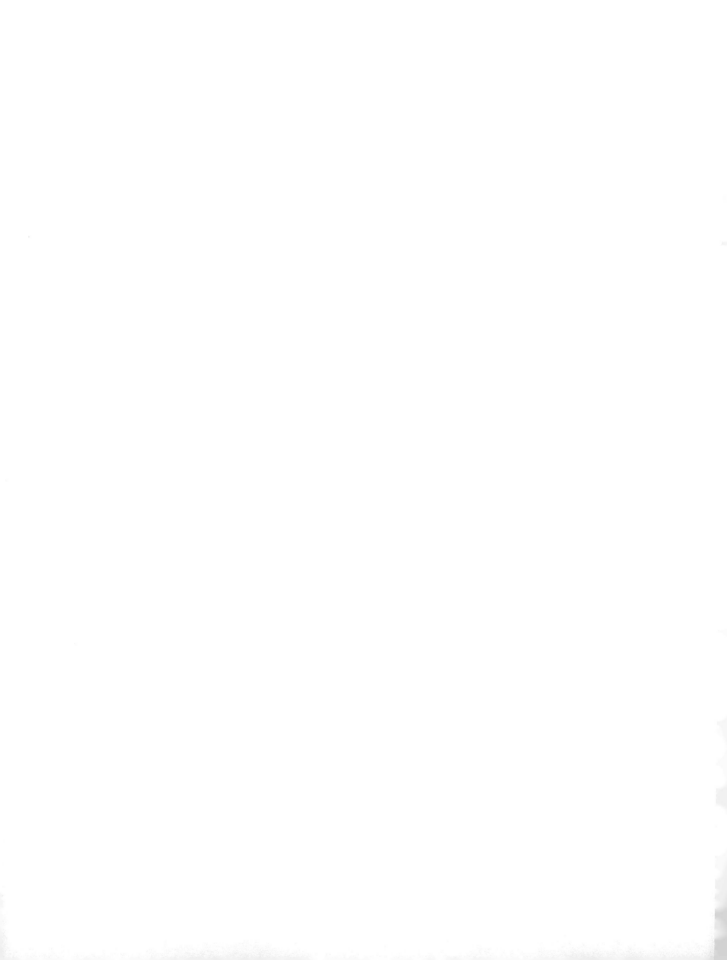

An Introduction to
Craniosacral Therapy
Anatomy, Function, and Treatment

An Introduction to
Craniosacral Therapy
Anatomy, Function, and Treatment

Don Cohen, D.C.

Illustrations by
Amie Forest and Jules Rodriguez

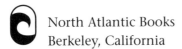

North Atlantic Books
Berkeley, California

Acknowledgments

To Karen, for everything

To John Upledger, for your teaching

To Deirdre Morrissey Scholar, for your tireless work on this
manuscript, and your wise and always valuable insight

To Jon Schreiber, for connecting and support

To Mark Bernhard, for research assistance

To Richard Grossinger, for seeing it through

To Jules Rodrigues and Amy Forrest, for your great illustrations

Thank you.

Published by
North Atlantic Books
P.O. Box 12327
Berkeley, CA 94712

Cover art by Amie Forest and Jules Rodriguez
Cover and book design by Leigh McLellan
Printed in the United States of America

An Introduction to Craniosacral Therapy: Anatomy, Function and Treatment is sponsored by the Society for the Study of Native Arts and Sciences, a nonprofit educational corporation whose goals are to develop an educational and cross-cultural perspective linking various scientific, social, and artistic fields; to nurture a holistic view of arts, sciences, humanities, and healing; and to publish and distribute literature on the relationship of mind, body, and nature.

North Atlantic Books' publications are available through most bookstores. For further information, visit our website at www.northatlanticbooks.com or call 800-733-3000.

ISBN-13: 978-1-55643-183-8

Library of Congress Cataloging-in-Publication Data

Cohen, Don.
     An introduction to craniosacral therapy : anatomy, function, and treatment / Don Cohen.
         p.   cm.
     Includes bibliographical references and index.
     ISBN 1-55643-183-X
     1. Craniosacral therapy.   I. Title
     [DNLM: 1. Osteopathic Medicine—methods.   2. Cerebrospinal Fluid.
     3. Central Nervous System.   WB 940-C678i   1995]
     RZ399.C73C64   1995
     615.8'2—dc20
     DNLM/DLC
     for Library of Congress   95-48203
                                                                      CIP

11 12 13 14 15   DATA   15 14 13 12 11

Contents

Contents

Contents

Fundamental Principles   68

Unwinding   82

Foreword

*T*he CranioSacral system is a core system in the human body. In my view it is the place where body, mind, and spirit reside independently and communally at the same time. By this I mean that the therapist (or better said, the therapeutic facilitator) can use either body, mind, or spirit individually, or the process can involve any combination of the three concurrently. Thus, the effect of the facilitative treatment process can manifest at almost any conceivable level from symptomatic relief to resolution of the very core problems of the spirit. The majority of times at least a significant combination of body and emotion is presented and treated. If the process is then pursued the spiritual realm will most often enter the scene and make its presence known.

It is this access to the very deepest problems that provides some of the uniqueness to CranioSacral Therapy. Another quality that makes this system of healing unique is that when properly administered by the CranioSacral therapist, the patient or client sets the agenda and guides the process. By this I mean that the CranioSacral Therapist tunes in to the inner wisdom and bodily intelligence of the patient or client and follows the plan of facilitative treatment put forth by this inner wisdom. This type of connection or rapport between patient/client and facilitator/therapist makes for a bond of mutual trust and love between the participants that often evolves into a healing, rather than a curing, type of resolution to presented problems and their underlying causes.

It is quite fascinating to consider that all of this very deep work is done within the confines of an anatomically defined physiological system. It suggests that the CranioSacral system and the techniques involved in CranioSacral Therapy offer a bridge between objective science and spiritual healing. Therapists who have become deeply involved in this system of patient/client interaction almost invariably report a deepening in their spiritual life and a strengthening of their emotional stability and sense of self worth.

The ultimate goal of CranioSacral Therapy is to free the patient/client from dependence upon any type of healthcare provider. Visits to healthcare providers would be for advice and for the facilitation of self-healing when the process encounters an obstacle that requires some help in overcoming. The patient/client only comes for help in the self-healing process, not for "curing" in the sense that the therapist "fixes" them. Thus, CranioSacral Therapy accesses the total human being's self-corrective and self-healing processes. Further, this therapeutic approach attempts to maximize patient/client responsibility for their overall well being.

Don Cohen has done an excellent job of presenting an overview of the various diagnostic, evaluative, and therapeutic approaches to the cranium, the sacrum, the dura matter envelope, and the fluid which it encloses. He is one of those rare individuals who has a real and true sense of the human body and what it is about. He also has a deep appreciation of the fact that the human body is not living in isolation. He knows both intellectually and intuitively about the interrelations between spirit, mind, and body.

John E. Upledger, D.O., O.M.M.
Palm Beach Gardens, Florida

Why Craniosacral?

*A*s a chiropractor, I was trained to consider the structure of the nervous system. Chiropractic teaches that healing is inherent and that our job is to remove interference to neurologic function. But my education and early practice raised more questions than they answered. What is the relationship between structure and function? What is the function of the nervous system? The craniosacral model, derived from osteopathy, sheds considerable light on these riddles.

This book was originally conceived and produced as a teaching manual for chiropractic doctors to accompany a Continuing Education class that I taught for Palmer College of Chiropractic West in Sunnyvale, Sacramento, and Los Angeles, California. While revising the book for the general public, I decided to leave intact many of the references to chiropractic concepts and philosophy that relate directly to those I discovered while working with the craniosacral system, as these concepts are universal and can be appreciated by non-chiropractors as well.

The word chiropractic means "hands-on." Traditionally, chiropractors have applied our hands to the spine because it represents a bridge between the brain and the rest of the body. But there are other conduits between these two systems as well. The craniosacral system offers us the opportunity to work directly with the cranial nerves, including the spine's quiet counterpart, the vagus, as they exit the foramina of the skull. In this way we can also more directly interact with the special senses. It offers a pre-foraminal approach to the spinal cord and nerve roots. And most importantly, the craniosacral system allows us to directly perceive and influence the structural configuration of the brain itself in its relationship to the body architecture, and gives us hands-on access to the interface between body, mind, and emotion. For those of us who subscribe to the unity of structure and function, this represents a significant opportunity.

The craniosacral system is the structural aspect of the central nervous system. It represents a "big picture" view that allows us to consider the behavioral aspects of the CNS organ and its manifestations throughout the body. It includes all of the structural components of the spinal subluxation concept and helps to shed some light on the nature of that phenomenon.

In this book we will consider the physiologic aspects of the nervous system and offer a simple, direct, and non-dogmatic whole-body approach to working with it that ideally will serve as a point of departure for accessing the inherent intelligence of our patient in a fluid and spontaneous way.

Since John Upledger taught me to listen to the organism with my body, my life has never been the same. This book is presented in the spirit of developing greater awareness of this enlightening mode of communication with the autonomic self.

The Fluid Medium: CSF

Cerebrospinal fluid (CSF), the fluid habitat of the central nervous system, is a highly specific fluid for the most sensitive organ. It is the role of CSF to provide the environment that is best suited for the survival and proper function of the brain and spinal cord, the body's main coordinating system. Should the CSF fail to serve its function within its extremely narrow parameters, irreversible damage and death ensue within minutes.

The central nervous system (CNS) is the body's most protected structure, the treasure in the citadel, and it's no mere coincidence that it occupies the structural core of the higher life forms. Encased within the armor of skull and spinal column, fortified by ligament and muscle, the central nervous system is a semi-closed-system environment, guarded by the exquisite mechanism of the blood brain barrier, a system of highly specialized tissues which, due to their specific permeability, effectively sequester CSF circulation from the other fluid systems of the body (i.e., blood, lymph, extracellular fluid) while allowing selective essential communication with them. CSF is emitted by the secretory cells of the choroid plexus and other central nervous system (CNS) tissues and circulates throughout the CNS in an ordered, one-way pathway, eventually being resorbed by the arachnoid villi of the sagittal sinus and returned to the blood venous system. It is, in a sense, a rarified, potentized refinement of the life-fluid, with its guardians at its gate.

Some History

The inquiry into the nature of the clear, colorless, odorless fluid observed in and around the brain dates back many centuries. The ancient Chinese medical classic, the *Ling-shu* (Ch'ing dynasty, 3rd century B.C.), makes fairly accurate reference to CSF, although it makes no distinction between it and extracellular fluid:

> When the refined fluids of the Five Cereals blend harmoniously, they constitute a Kao (lubricant) that is washed into the empty spaces of the bones and also replenishes the brain and medulla.

Galen (2nd century A.D.) observed the ventricles and believed them to be filled with air. European physicians at the dawn of the scientific age (16th century A.D.) were uncertain as to whether the water they observed in and around the brain and spinal cord in cadavers was present during life. Versalius in 1543 described the anatomy of the ventricular system which houses the CSF and noted the presence of a "watery humour" that often filled it. Descartes in 1664 described a model of fluid circulation from the heart to the cerebral cavities and then through the nerves to the muscles. Through this route, controlled by the pineal gland, flowed the "animal spirits," which were thought to flow through the nerves as a fluid circulation. Cotugno in 1764 first described the subarachnoid space, also comparing the "water" to that which fills the pericardium (ECF).

The continuity of the ventricular and subarachnoid fluid was established by Magendie in 1825 when he identified a foramen through the brain stem between the fourth ventricle and the subarachnoid space. It was on the basis of this knowledge that Magendie coined the term "Cerebro-spinal Fluid" in 1842. Magendie devoted his career to the study of the anatomy, physiology, and chemistry of CSF. His chemical analysis was remarkably good for the first half of the nineteenth century. Magendie is also on record as being the first to tap the cisterna magna of a living animal. Through these studies he correctly assumed that the CSF is constantly replenished.

In 1855 Luschka identified the two lateral foramina connecting the fourth ventricle with the subarachnoid space. Luschka also confirmed the theory of Faivre (1854) concerning the secretory nature of the choroid plexus in the production of CSF. This theory was still actively disputed as late as 1963 but is now universally accepted in the scientific community.

The last fifty years have seen tremendous advances in the accumulation of information regarding the anatomy, physiology, and chemistry of the cerebrospinal fluid system.

Much of the research into the applied physiology of the cerebrospinal fluid system has been rooted in intuitive understanding and clinical experience, the source of many breakthroughs in science.

Anatomy Of The Cerebrospinal System

The cerebrospinal fluid circulates around the brain and spinal cord in the sub-arachnoid space (external CSF) and within the brain and spinal cord in the fluid compartment comprised of the ventricles, the cisterna, the central canal of the spinal cord (internal CSF), and the various channels that connect these spaces.

The Meninges and Subarachnoid Space

Three concentric membranes, collectively known as the meninges (Latin: membrane) surround the CNS. The dura mater is the outermost of the meninges and forms a dense connective tissue envelope around the CNS. The pia mater, which intimately hugs the contour of the brain and spinal cord, is the innermost of the meninges. It extends into the spinal cord as septa, forming compartments. Between these membranes is a transparent sheath, the arachnoid, stretched over a delicate layer of reticular fibers, the arachnoid trabeculae, and forming a weblike membrane which extends medially to the pia. The arachnoid and pia are grouped as the leptomeninges ("delicate membrane") because they are functionally and microstructurally unified.

The space between the arachnoid and pia, filled with trabeculae and cerebrospinal fluid, is called the subarachnoid space. The subarachnoid space also delivers the arterial vessels to the brain. These vessels enter the substance of the brain, taking the arachnoid and pia mater with them and creating the perivascular space, an extension of the subarachnoid space which tapers as it

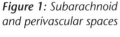

Figure 1: Subarachnoid and perivascular spaces

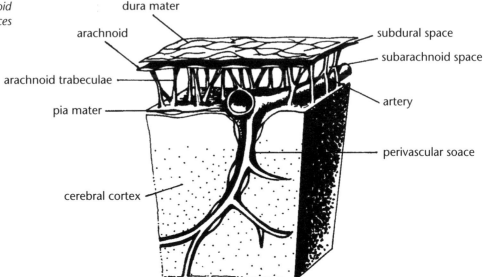

invaginates into the brain tissue. Thus the CSF circulation penetrates into the cerebral parenchyma (neurons and neuroglia).

The Subdural Space

Between the dura and arachnoid is a fluid-filled space. These membranes are not adherent but are freely gliding and filled with a watery fluid. The subdural space provides the venous drainage of the brain, also draining the spent CSF via the bulk flow through the arachnoid villi. The subdural space and the subarachnoid space are in equilibrium via pressure gradients.

The Cisterns

In certain areas the pia and the arachnoid are widely separated, creating CSF-filled meningeal sacs called **cisterns**. At the base of the brain and around the brain stem are the subarachnoid cisterna. Between the medulla and the cerebellum is one of the largest cisterns, the cerebellomedullary cistern or cis-

Figure 2: CSF spaces and cisterns

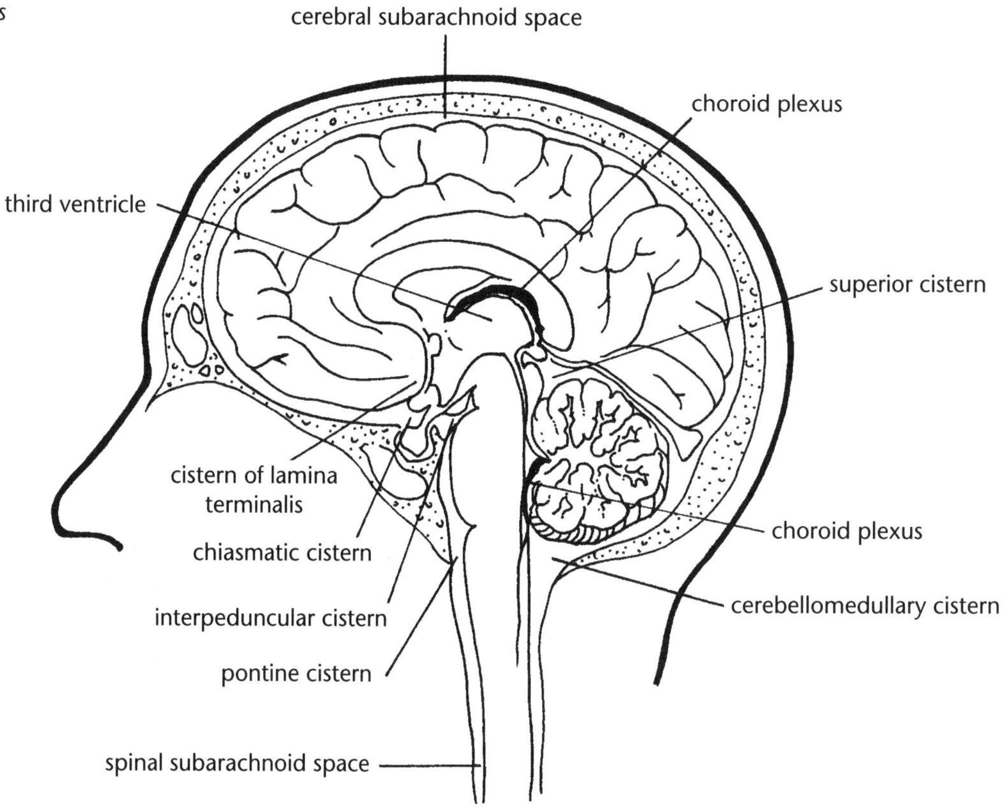

terna magna, into which the foramina of the fourth ventricle open (see previous page). Other cisterns of significant size are the pontine cistern, the interpeduncular cistern, the chiasmatic cistern, and the superior cistern or cisterna ambiens. At the base of the spinal cord is the lumbar cistern, which extends from the conus medularis to the level of the second sacral vertebra. It contains the 32 nerve roots (L3-S5 bilaterally) of the cauda equina ("horse's tail") of the spinal cord as well as the filum terminale. It is from this cistern that CSF is withdrawn in a lumbar spinal tap.

The Ventricles

The central nervous system in embryogenesis develops as a hollow tube, the notochord, and this concept is preserved in the mature CNS. In the center of the spinal cord is the central canal, which broadens out cephalically within the brain, forming a system of specialized hollows, the ventricles. The ventricles are laid out in a three-dimensional T-formation (see figure). There are two lateral ventricles, the largest and most complex in shape of the brain ventricles. Their arched, ram's-horn shape conforms to the general shape of the cerebral hemispheres which they inhabit.

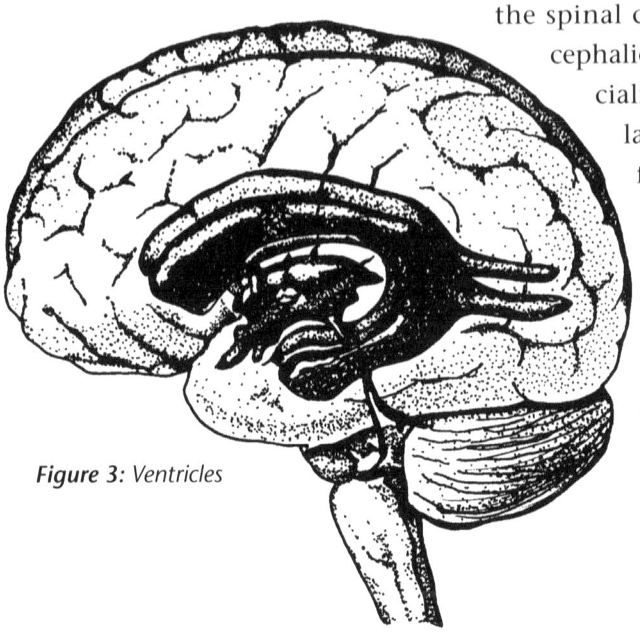

The lateral ventricles can be divided into five parts:

Figure 3: Ventricles

1. the anterior horn
2. the ventricular body
3. the collateral trigone
4. the inferior (temporal) horn
5. the posterior (occipital) horn.

Each lateral ventricle communicates with the narrow, midline third ventricle by the interventricular foramina of Munro. The fourth ventricle, also on midline, is broad and shallow, a rhomboid-shaped cavity overlying the pons and medulla and extending superiorly from the central canal of the upper cervical spinal cord to the cerebral aqueduct of Sylvius. The aqueduct of Sylvius communicates between the third and fourth ventricles. In addition, three small apertures exist at the caudal aspect of the fourth ventricle: the midline foramen of Magendie and two lateral foramina of Luschka, which communicate with the subarachnoid space.

Our Liquid Core

The structural center of the chordate is the notochord, a hollow tube. The vestige of the notochord in the mature NS is the central canal. It is lined with cilia and filled with pressurized cerebrospinal fluid which circulates from caudal to cephalic.

It is characteristic of living organisms to expend energy to counter entropy, the natural tendencies of gravity, inertia, and disorder.

This is our core: CSF rising.

Choroid Plexus

In the roof of the ventricles is the choroid plexus, a specialized tissue formed by ependymal tissue growing in a field of vascularized pia mater. The function

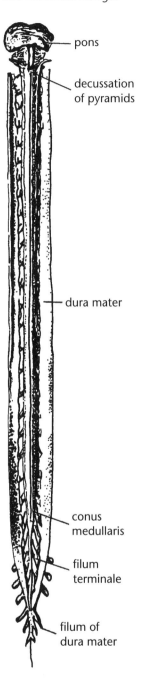

Figure 4: The spinal cord within the meniges

- pons
- decussation of pyramids
- dura mater
- conus medullaris
- filum terminale
- filum of dura mater

Figure 5: Choroid plexus tight junctions

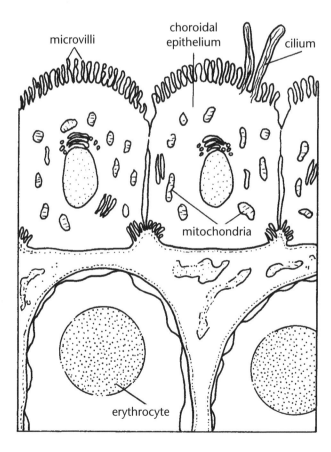

microvilli

choroidal epithelium

cilium

mitochondria

erythrocyte

of the choroid plexus is the secretion of CSF, with raw materials obtained from the arterial blood. The convoluted choroidal epithelium microvilli provide approximately 200 square cm of surface area which relieves the choroidal capillaries of about 25% of their plasma water in response to the osmotic gradient created by the active transport of Na+ into the CSF. About 500 ml of CSF is secreted by the choroid plexus daily, enough to turn over the body's contents four times. The choroid plexus is well supplied with extravascular nerve fibers that control secretion and others which closely resemble the Meissner corpuscle and probably have sensory function.

Figure 6: The three types of tissue capillary

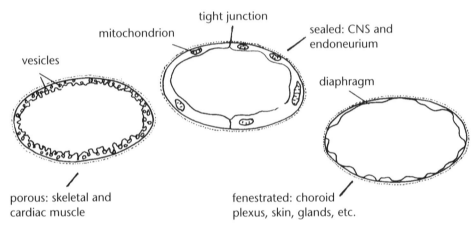

Blood Brain Barrier (BBB)

Critical to the concept of the CSF as a special fluid is the concept of the Blood Brain Barrier. The BBB is a general term used to describe what is actually a system of three barriers: blood-brain extracellular fluid (capillary endothelium), blood-CSF (choroid, etc.), and ECF-CSF (meninges). These barriers effectively sequester the CSF circulation from the blood and tissue ECF. Excepted from this fluid sequestration is the hypothalamus, which is the brain's "sensory organ" to the subtleties of the body fluids, and therefore lets them in.

The composition of CSF is strictly regulated by the combined efforts of the BBB and the choroid plexus. The anatomical basis for the BBB is believed to exist at the level of the brain endothelial cells that line the capillaries. The endothelial cells of capillaries in the brain differ ultrastructurally from those in muscle in that those in the brain have tight junctions (zona occludens, zo) rather than macula adherens (ma) between the cells. The macula adherens allows the easy passage of macromolecules from the blood into the tissue spaces

(ECF). Tight junctions restrict this passage. The cerebral capillary is further sealed by a discontinuous sheath of hydrophobic astrocytic foot processes (ap), which are interposed between blood vessels and neurons.

> "The barrier system stabilizes the physical and chemical milieu of the CNS and keeps highly sensitive neural elements in semi-isolation despite a rich blood supply." (Carpenter)

Equally strategic to the concept of the BBB is its permeability to essential elements. The brain must be provided with a steady-state level of energy, raw materials, ions, and oxygen in the proper concentrations, similar to a function of the carburetor in a combustion engine. The neurons are unforgivingly sensitive to deviations in the composition of CSF/brain ECF. The BBB performs this "carburetor" function via specific active transport and feedback mechanisms. CNS capillaries contain ten times more mitochondria than those of skeletal muscle, indicating significant metabolic activity.

Formation of CSF

The choroid plexus is a cauliflower growth of blood vessels covered by a thin coat of epithelial (ependymal) cells. It projects into the temporal horns of the lateral ventricles, the posterior portion of the third ventricle, and the roof of the fourth ventricle. CSF continually exudes from the surface of the choroid plexus via a complex of mechanisms. The choroidal epithelium contains a number of enzymes which facilitate ion transport across the BBB. Na+/K+/ATPase in the microvilli assists in the movement of Na+ into the CSF and K+ into the plasma. This in turn pulls negatively charged ions (especially Cl-) into the CSF as well, causing hypertonicity of the CSF. The osmotic gradient thus created causes large quantities of water and dissolved substances to pass through the choroidal membrane into the CSF. Water is also freely diffusible through the entire meningeal membrane. The composition of CSF is extremely specific. There are a number of other specific transport mechanisms active in the choroidal and brain capillary epithelia for monosaccharides, amino acids, electrolytes, etc.

Non-Choroidal Production of CSF

In addition to passing through the choroidal membrane, diffusion of water occurs freely between CSF and the blood vessels of the meninges. Also, diffusion and transport occur continually between CSF and the brain substance beneath the ependyma. The subarachnoid CSF contains metabolic water and electrolytes produced as waste products of cerebral metabolism and washed into the subarachnoid fluid in a one-way tendency from the lateral ventricles through brain tissue and the pia-glial membrane. This contribution to CSF is exempt from direct regulation by the BBB and accounts for less than 10% of CSF volume. Therefore, while it is true that CSF is continually produced by all CNS epithelium, the choroid produces the vast bulk of CSF and is responsible for the specificity of it, dwarfing other production to the point of being negligible.

Composition of CSF

Many of the constituents of CSF are remarkably independent of their concentration in the plasma. CSF differs from its source in electrolyte composition and the fact that CSF is relatively protein-free. Also there are no cellular components and few macromolecules. The BBB is designed to feed the CNS only the end-product elements refined from the metabolism of food. For these reasons CSF is classified as a secretion rather than as a simple filtrate. It is, of course, mostly water, with some dissolved elements:

1. **Glucose:** This is what the brain eats. The levels are below those of ECF. The brain will sacrifice a lot of body function to keep its soul-food levels consistent.

2. **Monocarboxilic acid**

3. **Amino acids:** Amino acids are transported across the BBB by one of three carriers according to their status as acidic, neutral, or basic. There is competition within each class for the carrier molecules; thus dietary or supplementary intake can influence which amino acids are able to cross the barrier into CSF. The amino acid tryptophan, for example, does not ionize at normal blood pH and competes with five other similarly neutral amino acids. Tryptophan is the precursor in the brain's synthesis of serotonin, one of the six well-established neurotransmitters. A decrease in the amount of tryptophan to the brain results in a similar decrease in the amount of serotonin synthesized in the brain. An increase in the provision of tryptophan may contribute to the competitive inhibition of another neutral and much-needed amino acid.

4. **Nucleic Acids:** These include specific carriers for adenine and nucleosides.

5. **Choline (amine)**

6. **Hormones**

7. **Vitamins:** B vitamins are especially prevalent.

8. **Electrolytes:** The brain electrolyte balance is also a delicately maintained homeostasis.

CSF Ions

The BBB contains numerous homeostatic mechanisms which protect the ionic composition of CSF from fluctuations in the rest of the body, including tight junctions, pressure gradients, and transport mechanisms. The CSF is in free equilibrium with the cerebral interstitial fluid, the unwavering composition of which is vital to the maintenance of the functional integrity of the brain. The homeostatic processes differ with each of the major ions, and in some cases the detailed mechanisms of these processes have not been worked out. They include active transport by the choroid epithelium as well as exchanges and transport at extrachordal sites.

Sodium (Na+) is the most abundant ion in CSF, ECF, and plasma, accounting for 95% of the total cation in these fluids. Other major CSF electrolytes are K+, Ca++, Mg++, and Cl-, as well as bicarbonate ion.

Conductive Medium

The electrical nature of the CNS is well known. One of the major roles of the CSF ions, especially Na, K, and Ca, is facilitating rhythmic electrical activity and the generation and delivery of the action potential in the CNS. This activity is basic to neurologic (and therefore all) function.

Some Other CSF Values

Volume: 150 ml
Specific gravity: 1.007
pH: 7.35
Chlorides (NaCl): 120-130 mEQ/l
Glucose: 65 mg/100 ml
Gamma Globulin: 6-13%
Total protein (amino acids):
    Lumbar: 15-45 mg%
    Cisternal: 10-25 mg%
    Ventricular: 5-15 mg%
      (from Chusid)

Drugs, Chemicals, and Toxins in CSF

Regulation of chemical entry into the CNS is governed by four factors:

1. **Lipid solubility:** Cerebral capillary (BBB) permeability to nonelectrolytes is governed by transendothelial diffusion and is therefore proportional

to lipid solubility. Due to its structural nature (lipid membrane), the BBB is especially effective against polar, charged, and hydrophilic substances. Highly lipid-soluble substances more easily pass through the barrier: anesthetics, caffeine, nicotine, steroids, the psychoactive drugs, and to a lesser degree, alcohol. Most antibiotics are weakly lipid-soluble and therefore require massive doses to be effective in the CNS.

2. **Ionization:** Only substances that are non-ionized at plasma pH (7.4) may pass the BBB. This mechanism blocks the entry of penicillin into the CSF.

3. **Plasma protein binding:** Many chemicals circulate in the blood bound to plasma albumin. The BBB is effective against these substances proportional to their degree of protein binding.

4. **Active transport mechanisms** determine the exceptions to the above factors.

The Blood Brain Barrier and Neurotransmitters

The BBB effectively sequesters the CNS transmitters (serotonin, etc.) within the meningeal envelope (they are recycled) and keeps non-CNS transmitters (epinephrine, norepinephrine, acetylcholine, dopamine) out of CSF, where they would wreak havoc. The CNS does lose a percentage of its neurotransmitters via pia-glial diffusion, along with metabolic water drainage through the bulk flow of CSF into the arachnoid granulations in the superior sagittal sinus.

The Blood Brain Barrier and Pathogens

The blood brain barrier is quite effective against most blood and extra CNS tissue pathogens and is equally effective against the body's immune response to pathogenic conditions within the meningeal envelope. For this reason CNS inflammation is often fast-acting and fatal and should be considered a dire medical emergency.

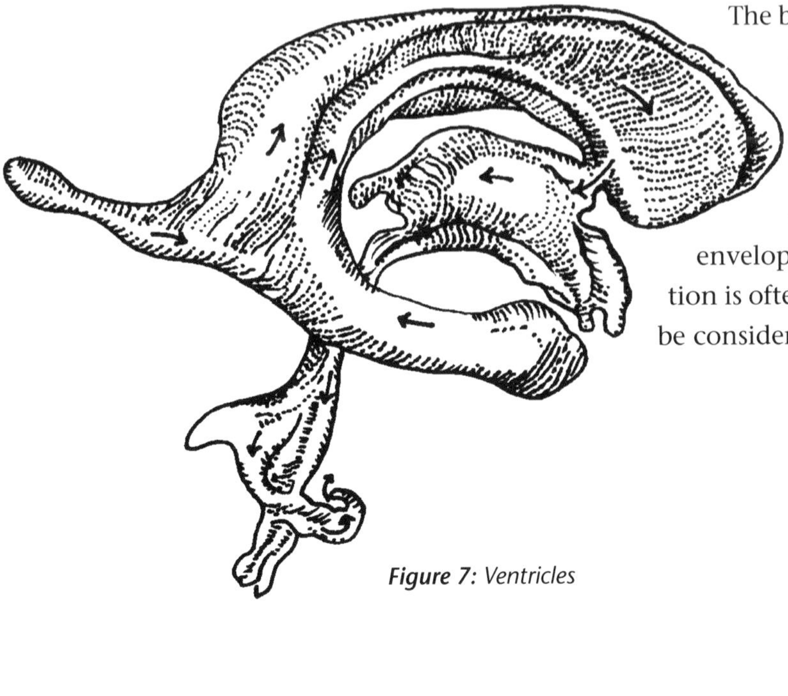

Figure 7: Ventricles

The Arachnoid Villi

The arachnoid villi (granulations) are specialized cauliflower-like structures that act as pressure-dependent one-way valves for the "bulk flow" of CSF out of the subarachnoid space into the superior sagittal sinus—a venous sinus created by a "splitting" of the falx cerebri where it forms a junction with the cranial dura, in the brain's midline cerebral fissure—in response to the pressure gradient between CSF and the venous blood system. This represents the endpoint of CSF circulation as it drains into the blood circulation. With a volume of 140 ml and a daily production of 500-700 ml, the CSF system exhibits significant daily turnover.

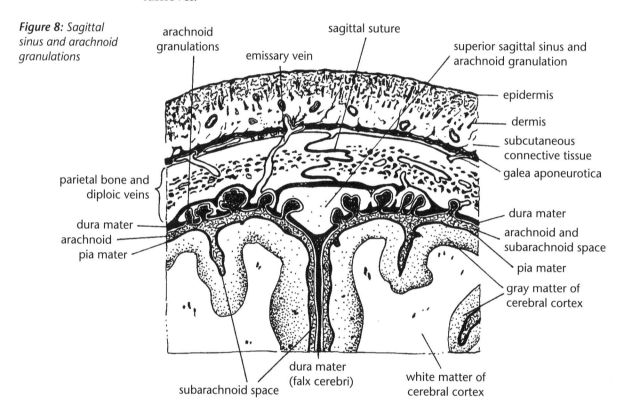

Figure 8: Sagittal sinus and arachnoid granulations

arachnoid granulations

emissary vein

sagittal suture

superior sagittal sinus and arachnoid granulation

epidermis

dermis

subcutaneous connective tissue

galea aponeurotica

parietal bone and diploic veins

dura mater
arachnoid
pia mater

dura mater

arachnoid and subarachnoid space

pia mater

gray matter of cerebral cortex

dura mater (falx cerebri)

subarachnoid space

white matter of cerebral cortex

Flow of Fluid in the CSF Fluid Space

Ninety-five percent of CSF is secreted by the choroid plexus in the lateral and third ventricles. Some of this fluid diffuses through the brain ECF to the subarachnoid space; the rest passes through the foramina of Munro into the fourth ventricle, where more fluid is formed. It next passes into the cisterna magna through two lateral foramina of Luschka and a midline foramen of Magendie.

Figure 9: *Flow of CSF*

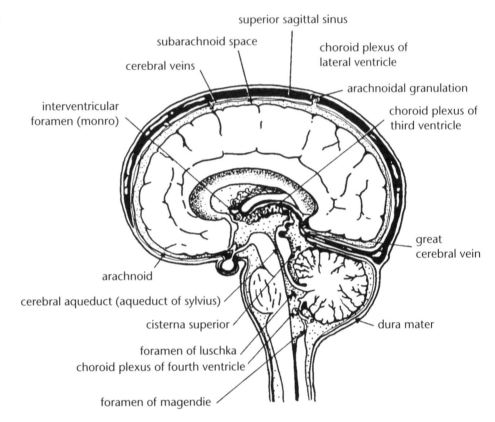

From here it flows through the subarachnoid space upward over the cerebrum and downward over the spinal pia. The subarachnoid space empties into the venous blood circulation via the arachnoid villi in the superior sagittal sinus, but first the CSF must pass through the small tentorial opening around the mesencephalon.

Diffusion Between CSF and the Ependymal and Meningeal Surfaces

The surfaces of the cerebral ventricles are lined with a thin cuboidal epithelium, the ependyma, and the CSF is in contact with this surface at all points. In addition, CSF in the subarachnoid space is in contact with the pia. The pia-glial and ependyma-glial membranes are freely permeable and diffusion occurs continually between the brain ECF and CSF. While the membranes are permeable, in both directions, there is directional net flow outward; ventricular (internal) CSF diffuses into brain ECF, and brain ECF diffuses into the subarachnoid space, joining the external CSF. In this manner the CSF continually washes through the brain parenchyma.

Brain Interstitial Fluid

Brain ECF is derived from both cerebrospinal fluid and the cerebral blood vessels, which deliver oxygen for the oxidation of glucose from CSF. The immediate milieu of the functional neuronal nuclei, brain ECF is in intimate equilibrium with CSF; they contribute to the composition of one another.

The brain ECF is the *in situ* environment of the CNS parenchyma and the direct mediator between the arterial (capillary) blood supply and the parenchymal cell. The two fluids—ECF and CSF—differ in composition mainly in terms of concentration of elements. The CSF serves as a conduit and reservoir of that which is vital to the function of the parenchymal cells.

Nutritive Function of CSF

The brain consumes glucose and oxygen. The internal and external CSF is in direct contact (via free diffusion into ECF) with the parenchymal cells of the cerebrum. The CSF functions as a primary conduit for some nutritive substances (especially glucose) and maintains equilibrium with the blood distribution of others, serving as a short-term reservoir for essential substances. The brain must be provided with a steady-state level of glucose in the proper concentration. It does not easily tolerate wide fluctuations in either direction: high brain glucose leads to diabetic coma, low brain glucose to insulin coma. The body will sacrifice its own tissues for the purpose of gluconeogenesis. In addition, the brain must be provided with the proper ions, vitamins, amino acids, etc.

"Lymphatic" Function of CSF

The one-way diffusion of CSF from the ventricles, through the brain parenchyma, and into the subarachnoid space washes metabolites (including metabolic water) into the external CSF. Also, a small amount of protein leaks out of the parenchymal capillaries into the interstitial spaces of the brain. Since no true lymphatics exist in the central nervous system, this protein, the waste products of CNS metabolism, and the wastes of brain immune function leave the tissues mainly through the perivascular spaces and by diffusion through the pia-glial membrane into the subarachnoid space, where they join with the CSF circulation and are eventually emptied into the superior sagittal sinus (venous blood) via bulk flow through the arachnoid villi.

Craniosacral work addresses this function directly, by encouraging the rhythmic action of the cerebrospinal system as it pumps the CSF through the brain tissue, replenishing the cells and draining the waste products of metabolism.

Figure 10: One-way CSF flow through the brain matter

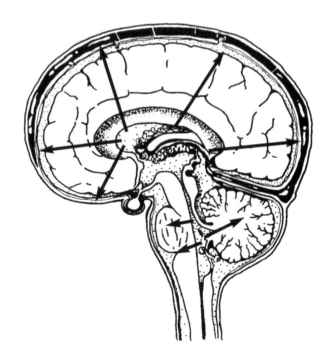

Hormonal Function in CSF

The "parietal eye," the pineal body, secretes into the third ventricle, communicating to other cerebral structures via CSF.

The Pieron Phenomenon

French physiological psychologist Henri Pieron suggested in 1913 that a substance may exist which is manufactured in the brain and circulates in the CSF, inducing sleep. Pieron transfused CSF from the cistern of sleep-deprived dogs to the CSF of rested dogs and noted that the recipients slept for several hours following the transfusion. The existence of sleep factor has also been reported by researchers at Harvard Medical School (1965).

CSF Pressure

The normal pressure in the subarachnoid CSF system is 130 mm H2O (10 mm Hg) recumbent (70-180 mm H2O is normal range). This is considerably greater pressure than the -6.3 Hg in the interstitial spaces of the rest of the body, and slightly greater than arterial pressure. CSF pressure is regulated by two factors: the rate of fluid formation and the rate of absorption at the arachnoid granulations. It is the fluctuation of these rates that is responsible for the fluctuation of the CSF pressure that we perceive as the cranial respiratory impulse.

Papilledema

The eyes are a direct extension of the brain, i.e., there is no synapse between the brain and the eye (or the nose). Anatomically the dura of the brain extends as a sheath around the optic nerve and then connects with the sclera of the eye. When the pressure rises in the CSF system, it also rises in the optic nerve sheath, causing the optic disc to swell. Papilledema is an important non-invasive diagnostic screen for pathologic conditions of the CNS.

The Labyrinthine Perilymph and Endolymph

The inner ear is contained within the petrous portion of the temporal bones. The **bony labyrinth** is constructed from bone which is harder and denser than that of the surrounding temporal bone, and it contains a fluid, the **perilymph**. Concentrically within the bony labyrinth and suspended in perilymph is the **membranous labyrinth,** and within it another secretion, **endolymph.** The motion and reaction to motion of these two fluids initiate the sensory functions of this cranial organ of spatial equilibrium. Two functional components of the labyrinthine structure sit side by side, sharing their fluid like Siamese twins:

1. The **vestibular mechanism,** with its semicircular canals, maintains equilibrium in conjunction with the visual apparatus via the cerebellum.

2. The **cochlea** translates sound vibrations into neural impulses.

In both components, endolymph is surrounded by perilymph, separated by a membrane. The ionic composition of the two fluids differs significantly. Endolymph, the only extracellular fluid with a high K+ concentration, more closely resembles intracellular fluid. Perilymph, a true ECF, has a higher concentration of Na+ and is continuous with the subarachnoid space via the perilymph duct through the temporal bone. Thus perilymph closely resembles CSF, and in fact is derived from it, with local secretion contributing as well. The ionic divergence of endolymph and perilymph contributes to a strong electrical potential gradient between them that facilitates the conversion of mechanical activity to electronic activity. This relationship serves both functions equally. Also of interest in this function are the otoconia, layers of calcium carbonate crystals embedded in a gelatinous layer covering the sensory maculae of the vestibular vestibule and in contact with the endolymph.

Projecting from the membranous labyrinth is the **endolymph duct,** extending like a pseudopod through a channel (the vestibular aqueduct) in the posterior petrous portion of the temporal bone and ending in a pouch, the

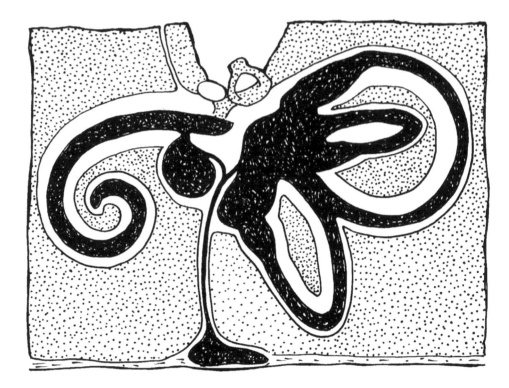

Figure 11: Membranous labyrinth

saccus endolymphaticus (**endolymph sac**), which enters through the external dura into the extradural space and rests against the internal dura. As well as providing bulk flow of the endolymph into the adjacent vascular plexus, this membranous dural window allows direct communication of pressure gradient and rhythm waves between the endolymph and CSF.

Relationship of CSF and Peripheral Nervous System

In theory, the CSF may wash freely through the peripheral nerve ECF because it is water and there is no barrier against it. Peripheral nerve ECF derives directly from the peripheral nerve capillary, which exhibits tight junctions and various transport mechanisms to provide a blood-nerve barrier. There is also a contribution by diffusion from the CNS interstitial fluid (and CSF), because there is no fluid barrier between them. This factor would, of course, decrease in more distal portions; peripheral pressure gradients probably favor the direct blood contribution in much of the PNS.

A microscopic space is found inconsistently between the peripheral nerve membranes. If there is a space, ECF will wash into it, and may then arbitrarily qualify as CSF as it is now between membranes.

Shock Cushion

Cerebrospinal Fluid is a hypertonic saline solution under pressure, with its specific gravity identical to that of brain tissue. The buoyancy it provides reduces the effective weight of a 1500-gram brain to about 50 grams. In addition, it provides an absorbent cushion against physical trauma to the cranium. Because the specific gravity of CSF and the brain are the same, blows to the head tend to move the entire brain simultaneously and distribute the force evenly, sparing any one portion of the brain the entire brunt of the force. In severe cranial trauma, the force of the blow can be transmitted like a whiplash through the fluid medium to the opposite side of the skull, bruising the brain on that side (contrecoup). The CSF is less effective in protecting the brain against violent rotational forces than it is against linear force vectors.

Sui-hai-ku: Brain Sea

Sui-hai-ku is an ancient Chinese concept. It means "Brain Sea" and refers to the occiput. It is a concept of the brain fluid that is almost startling in its allegory. The sea is a kinetic reference, ebbing and flowing, ubiquitous, enveloping, salty, prone to electrical storms, and full of myths, phantasms, and beasts.

The brain as it lies suspended in CSF is like a sea-creature, passively waiting in the depths, pumping and billowing, processing and waiting. It knows.

The Craniosacral Membrane System

The collagen membrane system contains the parenchyma of the body within individual fluid envelopes. As a tissue organ it exists in equilibrium with fluid pressure and exhibits "reciprocal conversion" with it—pressure into tension and tension into pressure. Through reciprocal tension it transmits the effects of these gradients to distal body parts, contributing to idiopathic symptomatology. This system of concentric and contiguous internal integuments surrounds virtually every anatomical component of the body—muscle and bone, neura and organ. The membrane can be seen as the skin of each body part, that which ultimately differentiates it from the surrounding tissue and fluids and expresses it as an entity. The ligaments, which bind the osseous levers, also qualify as collagen membrane. The connective tissue system, like all body systems, is highly organized and performs multiple simultaneous functions. The membrane system also contains and transports the meridian system.

Due to its anatomical, structural, and functional status, the craniosacral membrane system is referred to as the core membrane. It includes the falx cerebri, falx cerebelli, tentorium cerebelli, brain meninges, membranous labyrinth, and dural tube meninges. It is in reality one continuous membrane, like a semi-compartmentalized balloon, containing a highly specialized hydrostatic pressure system that extends down like a dipstick into the body from the cranium, existing in equilibrium with the tension and pressure of other body tissues and fluids.

Cranial Meninges

The brain meninges, discussed in the previous chapter, adhere to both the brain (pia-arachnoid) and the internal skull (dura). The cranial dura is bilaminal, with outer endosteal and inner meningeal layers, closely adherent except in specific areas where they separate to form venous sinuses. The endosteal layer which forms the periosteum of the inner skull adheres especially to the sutures (and is continuous with the sutural membrane), the cranial base, and the foramen magnum.

Figure 12: Cranial dura

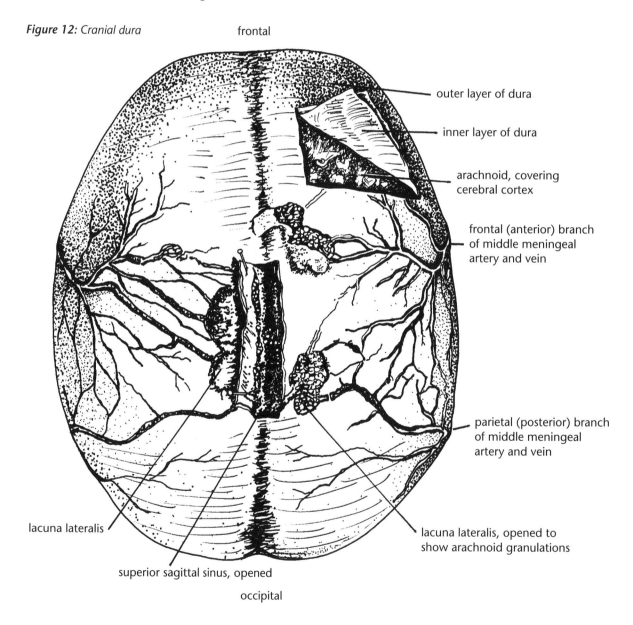

The cranial dura ensheathes the cranial nerves within their osseous foramina and fuses with each cranial nerve epineurium. It ensheathes the optic and olfactory nerves essentially in their entirety, fusing with the ocular sclera and providing a route for CSF to drain into the nasal cavities. It evaginates beneath the superior petrosal sinuses in the petrous temporal bone to form the cavum trigeminale, which encloses the trigeminal ganglion (sensory from the face). The clinical implications of these relationships are considerable.

Innervation of the Cerebral Dura Mater

The cranial dura receives both sensory and autonomic nerve fibers, mostly from the trigeminal nerve, the upper three cervical nerves, and the cervical sympathetic trunk. Sensory and proprioceptive nerve endings have been identified.

Figure 13: Meninges

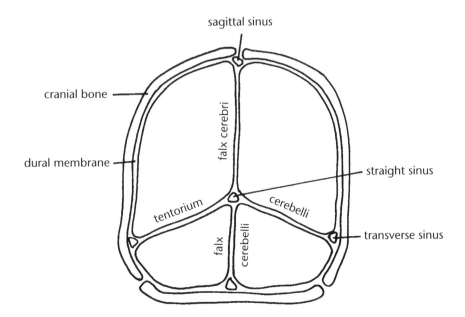

Intracranial Membranes

The meningeal layer of the cerebral dura invaginates into the matter of the brain, forming four septa which divide the cranial cavity, and the brain, into open compartments.

The sickle-shaped falx cerebri bisects the dome of the skull and the cerebral hemispheres through the sagittal plane (longitudinal fissure), arching over the corpus callosum. It is formed by an invagination of the cranial dura covering the right and left brain hemispheres, into the sagittal sulcus of the brain under the superior sagittal sinus. At its inferior border it splits once again to form the inferior sagittal sinus. The falx cerebri is narrow anteriorly and attaches to the crista galli of the ethmoid bone. Posteriorly it widens and blends with the tentorium cerebellum. At this junction is the straight sinus.

Figure 14: *Cranial membrane system*

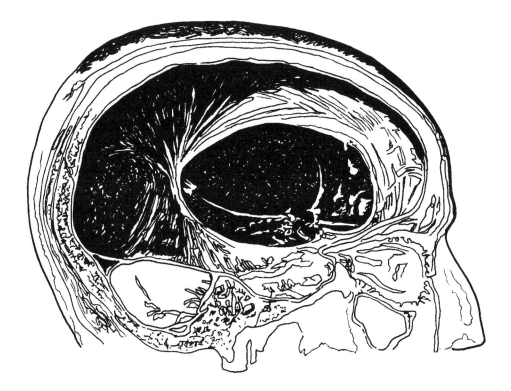

The horizontal tentorium cerebellum divides the occipital lobes of the cerebrum above from the cerebellum below. Its central free edge forms a crescent-shaped opening, the tentorial incisure, within which lies the midbrain. This central edge attaches anteriorly on either side to the anterior clinoid processes of the sphenoid bone. Here the oculomotor and trochlear nerves pierce the meningeal dura on their way to the eyes. Posteriorly, the peripheral tentorium attaches to the occipital and posterior-inferior parietal bones, containing the transverse sinuses, and laterally to the petrous portion of the temporal bones, where it contains the superior petrosal sinuses. It then blends with the dura and invaginates to form the recess of the cavum trigeminale, which encloses the sensory ganglion of the fifth cranial nerve. The peripheral tentorium then continues anteriorly to cross beneath its free border attachments and attaches bilaterally at the posterior clinoid processes of the sphenoid.

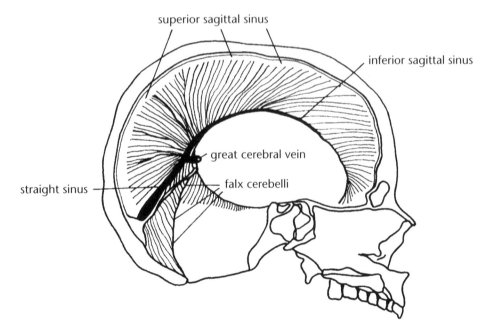

superior sagittal sinus

inferior sagittal sinus

great cerebral vein

straight sinus

falx cerebelli

Continuing beneath the straight sinus and tentorium cerebelli, the falx cerebelli shallowly divides the cerebellar hemispheres through the midline plane established by the falx cerebri. Its anterior free border arches around the vermis, the cerebellar analogue of the cerebral corpus callosum. Posteriorly it contains the occipital sinus, and inferiorly it attaches to the foramen magnum.

Lastly, the diaphragma sellae is a horizontal circle of dura which roofs the sella turcica and houses the pituitary, separating it from the optic chiasma. It is perforated by the infundibulum.

As you can see, each of the intracranial membranes is continuous with the meningeal dura and, through direct or reciprocal relationship, with each other. Each divides the brain matter into compartments while forming an opening through which important brain structures pass. They are fully innervated and also communicate cranial nerves and venous blood.

Dural Tube

The spinal meninges cover what Swedish neurophysiologist Alf Breig calls the "pons-cord tract." At the foramen magnum, the dura secures itself around the perimeter of the occiput and makes a short leap through the ring of the atlas to the spinal foramen of the second cervical vertebra. From there it cascades down the vertebral canal to the level of the second sacral segment, where it meets the coccygeal ligament, or filum terminale externum. From the second cervical vertebra to the second sacral segment the dura is relatively freely gliding, bound only by the nerve roots which carry it at right angles into each intervertebral foramen.

The Craniosacral Membrane: A Pump

The craniosacral membrane contains the brain's fluid milieu. Its structure allows elastic expansion to rhythmic pressure increase and offers a tensile rebound in its "diastolic" recovery, similar to the way nylon might respond. It therefore acts as a pump mechanism in conjunction with the cranial rhythmic impulse in the cerebrospinal fluid.

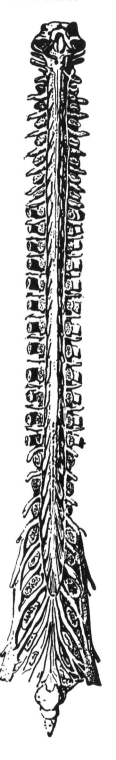

Figure 16: Cascade: the dural tube

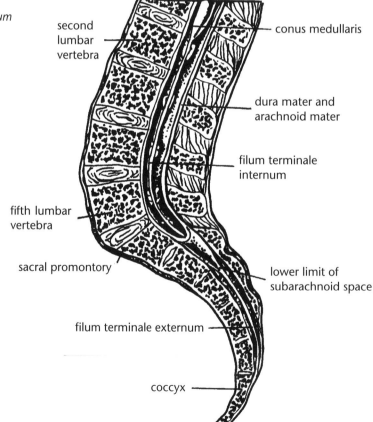

Figure 17: Filum terminale internum and externum

second lumbar vertebra

conus medullaris

dura mater and arachnoid mater

filum terminale internum

fifth lumbar vertebra

sacral promontory

lower limit of subarachnoid space

filum terminale externum

coccyx

The Dural Persona

The dura is the integument of the central nervous system. The fluid environment within it contains the constituent chemical and electrical nature of the brain parenchyma in intimate and unrestricted homeostatic equilibrium. More to the point, the membrane and the fluid it contains are the brain to the same degree as the parenchyma and the neuroglia. The persona of the individual human central nervous system, without exception the most expressive entity of creation-as-we-know-it, is expressed in the meninges in the same way that we identify a person at their "skin level." The skin ultimately defines the interface of self and not self (world). The dura is the skin, and therefore the persona, of the central nervous system. Distortion forces in it are transmitted directly and indirectly to the tissue of the brain.

The Craniosacral Skeleton

The craniosacral skeleton is the axial skeleton. It consists of the skull, vertebral column, sacrum, and coccyx. It is a neurologic skeleton. The traditional weight-bearing "chiropractic skeleton" excludes the skull, except for the occipital condyles, but includes the pelvis. The dynamic skeleton, of course, has both activities simultaneously.

The Skull

The skull can be divided into the **face** and the **calvarium.** There are 28 moveable bones in the craniofacial skull, including the six ossicles of the inner ears within the temporal bones. Additionally, and also within the temporal bones, are the **osseous labyrinths.** The **hyoid** bone is considered by some to be cranial. Lastly, the teeth reside in the skull and are subtly moveable.

There are eight cranial bones:

1. occiput
2. sphenoid
3. ethmoid
4. frontal
5. two temporals
6. two parietals

There are fourteen facial bones:

1. mandible
2. vomer
3. two maxillae

4. two zygomatic
5. two palatines
6. two nasals
7. two lacrimals
8. two inferior conchae

The Teeth

The teeth are craniofacial structures and can influence the craniosacral mechanism to a considerable degree. The individual teeth can be palpated for motility and can be adjusted by various means. They can also be adjusted as a whole (the bite). In addition, the dental arch is available as a lever on cranial mechanics via the palate.

The Sutures: Joints

The inevitable fusion of the adult skull has long been an accepted anatomical dogma. The craniosacral model refutes this concept as its basic premise, and instead presents a concept of the sutures as joints which retain integrity of motion throughout normal life. Like all joints, the undulating interdigitations of the cranial sutures are designed to facilitate certain motion and to restrict other motion, thus fulfilling the dual function of providing both stability and motility. Sutures are unique to the skull and are classified as fibrous joints. There are several types of sutures:

1. **Serrate sutures** are characterized by edges that interdigitate in a serrated fashion, with the teeth of the interdigitations tapering slightly. The sagittal suture is an example of this. This configuration allows gapping of the joint.

2. **Denticulate sutures** are similar to serrate sutures but exhibit a "dovetail" effect, with the teeth widening toward the ends, which more effectively locks the suture. The lambdoid suture is usually of this type.

3. **Squamous sutures** are characterized by overlapping bones, such as the temporal and parietal, which are reciprocally beveled. There are two types of squamous sutures: **limbous sutures** have mutual ridges or serrations, and the more common **plane sutures**, which exhibit less structured surfaces which are mutually roughened, such as the temporoparietal suture, the suture between the two maxillae, or the meeting of the zygomatic and palatine bones.

Gray's Anatomy, 39th British Edition, lists 34 cranial sutures, including the metopic suture, which is present in the neonate but normally fuses and disappears by the eighth year. It remains viable in a minority of adults.

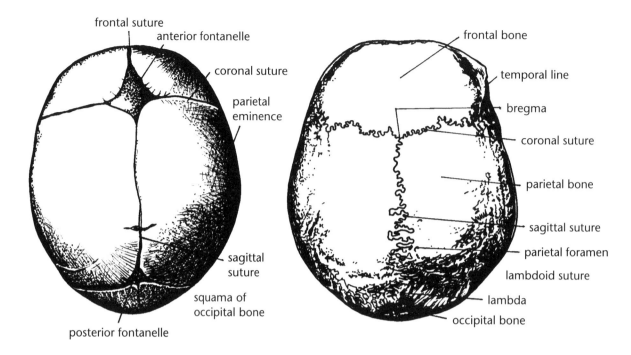

Figure 18: *Sutures, neonatal and mature*

The Orbits

Seven bones comprise each orbit; including shared midline structures, twelve bones join to form the two orbits. The advantage of this moveable design over that of the sella turcica (a hollow scooped out of a single solid bone) probably has to do with the advantages that a pump mechanism offers to the eye. The influence of craniosacral structural and hydraulic function on the eye is potentially significant.

Two bones are shared by both orbits:

1. frontal (called the orbital plate)
2. sphenoid, greater wings and lesser wings (orbital processes)

In addition, each orbit contains a contribution from each of the following:

3. maxilla (orbital plate)
4. zygomatic (orbital process)
5. palatine (orbital process)
6. ethmoid (orbital lamina)
7. lacrimal (posterior crest)

Adjustment of the orbits is achieved by mobilization of their components. The sphenoid, ethmoid, and palatine are not accessible in situ and must be influenced by lever mechanics from a distance.

The Palate

The roof of the mouth is formed by the maxillary, palatine, and vomer, and plugs into the anterior sphenoid. The palate can be adjusted intraorally, but this is not discussed in this text.

Figure 19: The palate

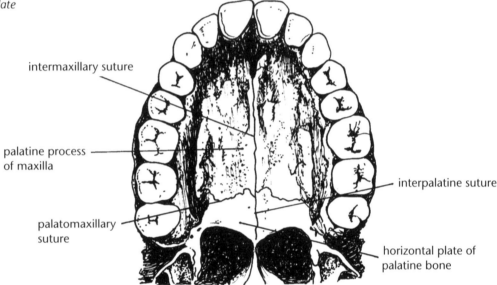

intermaxillary suture

palatine process of maxilla

interpalatine suture

palatomaxillary suture

horizontal plate of palatine bone

Caution: The orbits and palate are especially sensitive areas.

Any damage here may be disastrous. The application of force to the eye and palate has been associated with convulsive disorders. Avoid using undue pressure when working near the eyes or in the mouth.

The Sutural Ligament

Between the interdigitating surfaces of the cranial sutures is a connective tissue membrane, the sutural ligament. This soft tissue filler fulfills the requirement of providing cranial stability and also allows subtle motion between the cranial bones as a means of accommodating the rhythmic fluctuation of fluid pressure within the cranium. The sutural ligament contains vascular and neurologic elements.

Sutural Proprioceptive Mechanism

Upledger has identified in the monkey single nerve axons which he traced from the sagittal suture, through the meninges, and into the wall of the third ventricle. He theorizes that this may be evidence of a sutural proprioceptive mechanism which contributes to the control of rhythmic CSF production by the choroid plexus of the ventricles.

The Sutural Bones

The sutural bones are small, isolated, and irregular bones which may occur within sutures. They are thought to represent auxiliary ossification centers and occur most frequently within the lambdoid sutures, at the posterior fontanelle, and between the parietal bone and the greater wing of the sphenoid. While not uncommon in normal skulls, sutural bones are often found in frequent numbers in cases of hydrocephaly.

Mobilization of Sutural Restriction

Like all joints, the mobility of a sutural joint is limited by its shape. All types of sutures are prone to compaction and some degree of shear. There may be diverse torsional, side bending, or other forces imposed on the sutures by the attitude of the bones and the subosseous milieu, and they will express these forces as various forms of jamming according to their shape and circumstance. It is good to traction the sutures apart, and in addition they can be tractioned in relationship to the membrane system, which attaches to the underside of the bones and is responsible for much of the distortion. This is the orientation of the ten-step protocol presented later in this book. Lastly, "v-spread" (or "direction of energy") and "unwinding," two dynamic processes to be discussed, may be utilized with the sutures.

Practice: Sutural Proprioceptive Response (Sutural Spread)

The sutures can be tractioned manually with the thumbs or fingers. You can follow the course of all the sutures through the skull. You might begin with the temporoparietal sutures and then move the sagittal suture. There is evidence of proprioceptive nerve endings within the sutures, and Upledger suggests a possible relationship between the sagittal suture proprioceptive mechanism and the rate of production of CSF.

Blend your hand with your subject and use a gentle pressure, being certain to introduce pure traction without unwittingly compressing any other sutures. Proceed slowly and patiently. An understanding of the anatomical details of the various sutures will enable you to gain maximum benefit and avoid creating any unnecessary complications. You might notice that at certain points, the sutures will invite you to hold the traction for a bit, and perhaps some unwinding will occur between the bones as expressed in your fingers. When the unwinding has completed, continue to move along the sutures. You can also try pumping the sutures by gently and slowly tractioning and releasing them rhythmically.

I know of one case where a man who had been in a severe auto accident coincidentally emerged from several days of coma directly after sutural traction was applied.

Non-Sutural Cranial Articulations

There are two types of non-sutural joints in the skull. The perpendicular plate of the ethmoid fits into a groove in the vomer. The vomer in turn is ridged and fits into a groove in the rostrum of the sphenoid. These are both examples of a **schindylesis.**

Secondly, the teeth fit into the alveolar sockets of the mandible and maxilla and are held by fibrous periodontal ligaments. This type of joint is called a **gomphosis.**

Vertebrae

The vertebral system is a powerful and basic adaptive mechanism. The vertebrae segmentally armor the upright central nervous system from the tension, pressure, trauma, and gravitational pull of the body, and in doing so segmentally represent the demands of the body to the CNS, while protecting it from the immediacy of those demands. The nervous system reads the body configuration inherently, that is, autonomically and by virtue of itself.

It is agreed by all that the vertebral functions include armoring, mobility, and weight-bearing. Chiropractic understands that the vertebrae function neurologically as well.

The Atlas and Upper Cervical Mechanism

The upper cervical mechanism consists of the occiput and the first two cervical vertebrae (atlas and axis). It maintains strong structural and neurological individuality from the time of birth, being partially exempt from reliance on the postnatal development of myelin for its musculoskeletal function. The upper cervical relationship to the craniosacral system is discussed further in the dural tube chapter.

Sacrum and Coccyx

The sacrum and coccyx are the inferior component of the craniosacral system, providing attachment for the meninges. The sacrum provides the dual function of weight-bearing and craniosacral respiratory motion while also transporting the sacral and coccygeal plexuses. When healthy it provides an anchor for the meningeal tension and rhythm. Because it is the meeting place of weight-bearing (outgoing) and shock-absorbing (incoming) vectors with the neural function, proper sacral angle is an indication of uprightness, the expression of the upward urge of our central canal CSF core. The sacral angle is the structural base of lumbar lordosis and offers a healthy counter-response to the stress collapse of the spine towards the fetal kyphosis. The sacrum is discussed further in the chapters on the craniosacral rhythmic impulse and the dural tube.

The Pelvis

The pelvis is not a craniosacral structure, but as the seat of the sacrum it relates weight-bearing and shock-dispersion function to the craniosacral mechanism. Therefore, although not addressed directly in this text, pelvic balance can have a profound effect on craniosacral function.

The Craniosacral Rhythmic Impulse

The Fluid Model

The craniosacral rhythm is a brain-generated fluid pulse that emanates from the central fluid core structure (ventricles) outward. "From the inside out, from the top down." Upledger theorizes that the origin of the rhythm is the intermittent proliferation of CSF by the cells of the choroid plexus (the "pressurestat model"), and he has identified proprioceptive neurons from the sagittal suture to the ventricles which may control this function by feedback mechanism. As the choroid plexus function fluctuates, the CSF hydrostatic pressure also fluctuates, at a normal rate of six to ten times per minute. This pressure gradient wave drives the circulation of CSF rhythmically through the brain tissue from the ventricles outward to the subarachnoid space. Thus the choroid plexus is the "heart" of the brain. The CSF also circulates through the foramina and other ventricles and down to the base of the brain and into the subarachnoid space (SAS).

The pressure inside the ventricles is greater than that of both the brain extracellular fluid and the subarachnoid space. This pressure gradient contributes to both circulatory routes of CSF.

The cranial membrane-suture mechanism allows CNS pressure homeostasis by the rhythmic increase of volume in the cranial vault. The expansion and contraction of the cranial tissues, both hard and soft, is transmitted via structural tissue integrity through the nervous system and whole body. Because the body structure is repeatedly, down to microscopic levels, composed of two units, fluid and membrane, the rhythm is transmitted through the body by two mechanisms:

1. **Fluid wave transmission:** The body is 97% water. The wave is a moving pressure gradient through the fluid medium. To understand the phenomenon of rhythm in the body, consider that the whole thing is under water.

2. **Membrane tension:** Soft tissue membrane (fascia) will transmit a fluid wave but also tends to pull, and therefore offers resistance to gentle mobilization. Hard tissue (bone and cartilage) pushes. Bones act as levers and tend to act on other bones in a gear-like manner at the joints. The motion is pressure-driven, and the tissues that provide resistance also act through pressure and tension gradients.

Physiologic Motion: Motility

Physiologic motion is the motion inherent to life. All organisms and living functional units demonstrate inherent motion. Gross forms of physiologic motion include those of breathing, cardio-vascular rhythm, and peristalsis. There are also more subtle forms of physiologic motion. The unit of physiologic motility is the fluid-filled membrane sac, which exists repeatedly as a structural theme of the organism from the gross to the microscopic. Motile units include the whole body, fascial fluid compartments (including the meninges), organs within their capsules, cells, etc. Besides functioning as an expression of aliveness, physiologic motion plays a vital role in the movement of fluids throughout the body.

The Motile Effect of CRI on Neurons

This speculative functional model is offered as a possible explanation of the palpable phenomenon of the craniosacral rhythmic impulse (CRI) throughout the body, based on anatomic and physiologic concepts and on Upledger's idea that the choroid plexus functions intermittently through feedback mechanisms.

The brain is soft and gelatinous, and the spinal cord is only slightly firmer. Alf Breig remarks that CNS tissue acts as a fluid of low viscosity and displays the plastic property of deformation and the elastic property of recovery. The rhythmic force of the fluid wave from the ventricles through the brain parenchyme rotates the neuron nuclei like seaweed floating in the ocean. The neural fascicles carry the motion down the spinal cord as a slow, whip-like corkscrew wave, not passively but behaviorally. The CRI, generated bilaterally by the two lateral ventricles and by the bilateral pattern of the falx membrane, the brain and the body, represents the inherent motion (motility) of the neurons which is transmitted through the fluid and membrane structure of the viscera and the musculoskeletal system along the longitudinal axis. It has been noted that the CRI is not present in body structures that have been denervated— for example, when the spinal cord is severed.

The Phenomenon of Pulsation

The universe demonstrates biphasic activity of either binary (digital) or logarithmic (analog) wave form. All forms of electromagnetic, sonic, and life-process activity (energy) exhibit this phenomenon, on macro and micro levels.

The body exhibits polyrhythmic activity. The Electroencephalogram and Endocardiogram rhythms readily demonstrate this principle, as do the vascular and breathing functions. There are also myriad rhythms in various tissues and at different "levels." The craniosacral rhythm represents a slow, unifying wave pulsation through the tissues. The parallels to music are apparent. It is the organized subjective experience—conscious, "subconscious," and autonomic—of all rhythmic activity that allows us to function harmoniously. Disharmony and discord are also dysrhythmia. The harmony of all pulsation and signaling in the body is a subjective experience and cannot be deduced from the component parts. It represents the organism's overall ability to organize in counter to the tendencies toward entropy (stress). As an expression of adaptive reserve, or vitality, the CRI represents the harmony of function.

Normal Physiologic Motion: Flexion and Extension

The terms flexion and extension are used to designate the two phases of craniosacral respiration. Craniosacral flexion and extension bear no direct relationship to the approximation of flexor and extensor surfaces of the limbs and torso, but represent the "systolic" and "diastolic" phases of CSF production. There are approximately ten CRI cycles per minute, each cycle including one flexion and one extension phase. The two CRI phases can be palpated as a subtle urging motion in all the body's structural components: the cranium, the sacrum, and on the limbs and torso.

Cranial Flexion and Extension

The cranial vault and facial structures expand and contract in response to the fluctuation of the CSF pressure. The motion is subtle and its extent can be imagined from the observation of sutural range of motion, keeping in mind that the sutures are occupied by cartilage. The motion is felt as an impulse rather

Figure 20: Cranial flexion and extension (exaggerated)

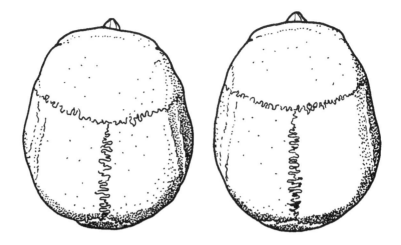

than a gross movement. In cranial flexion (choroid systole) the skull widens and shortens. In cranial extension (choroid diastole) the skull lengthens and narrows.

Sphenobasilar Mechanism

The junction of the sphenoid and the basilar portion of the occiput, just anterior to the foramen magnum, is the functional fulcrum of osseous cranial motion. The joint, a synchondrosis, acts as a subtle gear-hinge, with the sphenoid flexing anteriorward and the occiput flexing posterior.

The cranial base is closely associated with the spinal column because it evolves embryologically with the column from cartilage derived from the notochord. This has been traditionally interpreted to signify that the sphenobasilar hinge is the primary motivation of the CRI while the cranial vault, derived from embryologic membrane, simply accommodates the motion. The "pressurestat" model of fluid wave generation by the choroid plexus attributes the primary motivation of the CRI to non-osseous origins.

The embryogenesis of the cranial base as an intrinsic spinal structure emphasizes the relevance of cranial function to our work as chiropractors. The cranium is certainly the head of the spine.

Temporals

The design of the temporal bones provided the original inspiration for William G. Sutherland's concept of cranial bone motion. He noticed that the temporal sutures are "beveled like the gills of a fish" and the bones swivel around a rotatory horizontal axis in a spiraling fashion that in flexion flares the anterior

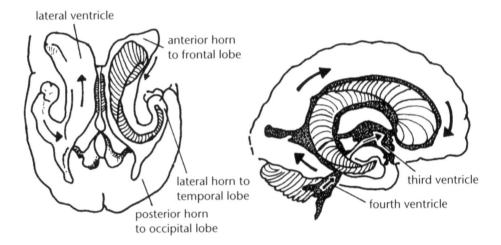

Figure 21:
Ram's horns

aspects laterally, like gills, and approximates the mastoids. The motion of the temporals reflects the "ram's horn" configuration of the lateral ventricles.

Sacral Flexion and Extension

There is a mild intermittant traction of the spinal dura with the phases of craniosacral rhythm. The sacral base rocks posterior (and the sacral apex anterior) with craniosacral flexion, and anterior (sacral apex posterior) with extension. Skilled palpation of this function can assist in the location of restrictions in the dural tube.

Whole Body Flexion and Extension

Craniosacral flexion urges each half of the body to subtly rotate laterally. Each limb also rotates along the longitudinal axis, externally with the flexion phase and internally with craniosacral extension. These changes can be palpated but usually cannot be observed visually; however, on occasion there will be visual clues, for example, in the case of a pigeon-toed child. If the hands are also turned in, the child may be fixed in craniosacral extension.

A more detailed account of osseous craniosacral motion can be found in the texts by Upledger and Magoun. These texts are listed in the Bibliography.

Physiologic Motion as an Indicator of Adaptive Vitality

The ease with which a tissue or an organism comfortably occupies its niche and moves freely within that space is an indication of the ability of the tissue or organism to function optimally. There are two implications of this phenomenon.

1. **Mobility** refers to movement, both active and passive, through a range of motion. There are numerous possible causes for any lack of mobility, among them chronic body use patterns, postural defects, extrinsic trauma, present or past inflammation, post-surgery, etc. Lack of mobility is most often a characteristic of membrane restriction (hard or soft) and may be either a "holding pattern" or a "breakdown" pattern. In most cases, chronic loss of mobility is characterized by the deposition of "cheap-grade" fiber, or adhesions.

2. Every organism and every tissue demonstrates inherent rhythmic motion. This is **motility**. Chronic challenge to any tissue or system may result in a long-term alteration of its motility. Lack of motility is a palpable representation of the system's struggle to function. Of course mobility and motility exert varying degrees of influence on one another.

The CRI represents the inherent motility of the central nervous system. When the CNS encounters input to which it must adapt or which requires change or the processing of new information (stress), it momentarily ceases to process its workload so as to integrate the input. This can be palpated as a pause in the motion of the unit, a shutting down of the CRI (a **still point**), which according to our model represents a suspension of the rhythmic choroid plexus production of CSF and often correlates with the changes detected by polygraph.

In palpating for craniosacral motion, observe the characteristics of the waveform and also the body's tendency to transmit or resist the impulse. Be curious as to the number of agendas that the organism is attending and the nature of these concerns. This represents a kind of overview in which we ascertain the extent to which the organism is functioning as a whole as represented by the impulse of the cranial rhythm and the ease with which the tissues accommodate it. A "local agenda" will offer resistance to both fluid wave transmission (rhythmic pressure gradient) and membrane gliding.

Picture a bubbling mountain spring cascading confidently and delightfully along. It fills up every nook and cranny in its course, always finding the path of least resistance to overcome every obstacle. In contrast, imagine a dammed-up and lazy river that winds through an industrial city in midsummer. Barely moving, its waters murky and thick, dusted with floating sediment and debris, and subject to stagnation and bacterial infestation, it presents a very different dynamic.

The Induction and Transmission of Wave Activity by Lesions

Any active or passive impairment may create a pattern of interference in the rhythmic field and tensile balance of the body. Energetic (behavioral) malfunctions create wave motion in the fluid medium which interferes with the physiologic motion, like a reed blown by the wind, superimposing its interference pattern in the rhythmic medium of a lake.

The World of Rhythm

The craniosacral rhythm is one player in an ensemble. The entire ensemble plays a number in which the exact melody may be hard to define. We seek a broader metaphor. Place your hand on a back or chest or belly. Blend your hand, fluid into fluid. "Rhythmos" means fluid. Focus on the craniosacral rhythm, then expand your focus. Let the hand float and listen to the whole body rhythm without expectation. All of the body rhythms—craniosacral, cardiovascular, respiratory, bioelectrical, adaptive (interference), and a myriad of others—are occurring simultaneously. This is holism. It's rather like the ocean in the way the whole thing ebbs and flows; there's a rhythm but there doesn't seem to be an exact pattern. This "sum of the parts" palpation is a good spot for fishing.

The Clinical Significance of the Craniosacral Rhythm

Stress is a whole-system response read most effectively "not as a sum but as an integral." With this in mind our interest is in the integrated subjective status of our patient as perceived in his or her nervous system by our nervous system. The craniosacral rhythm represents the "big picture" status of the brain attitude and serves as a tuning device for the long-loop function. Give yourself permission to feel and use it to plug in. You may choose to focus on the rhythm, or may instead shift your focus to tension, lever, and pressure forces in the body, moving freely between aspects, registering the impression as you go. Imagine that you can get an image of the patient's body in your somatic cortex. With practice this tuning process will become second nature and occur more quickly.

The craniosacral rhythm also lends clues to the significance of the process occurring at any given time. It stops to integrate change and pumps along when things are status quo. This helps in assessing the potential benefit should we consider exploring any avenue. The nervous function is innately interested in gaining homeostasis and will pause for each potential lightening of the burden that it lugs around. If no change is likely you'll not want to waste time with an issue.

It's natural for some of us to resist this kind of free-form association. Our culture is suspicious of subjectivity and frowns on it severely. We're vigilant against being hoodwinked and maintain our objectivity as our defense. On the other hand, total objectivity limits us to the five senses, leaving us detrimentally estranged from our own selves, stranded on the desert island of biologic technology, where health and disease are entities and not a process.

As the world quickens, our process quickens as well. If we trust it, the worst thing that can happen is nothing. If we don't, the worst thing that can happen probably will.

The History of the Craniosacral Concept

*I*t was the dogged determination of one man, William G. Sutherland, D.O., that brought the craniosacral concept through from a flash of insight to our present recognition of this vital concept of central nervous system behavior. Without his vision and tenacious perseverance, the concept would have withered and perished from scorn.

Ebb and Flow

In 1929 a German psychiatrist named Hans Berger was angered by the failure of the scientific community to recognize the significance of his work. In that year he published some pictures consisting of nothing but little squiggles. Berger's claim to have demonstrated graphic proof of the brain's electrical activity was not taken seriously, in great part due to the attitude prevalent at the time that it was not really respectable to study the activity of the brain with measuring instruments. In fact, Berger did demonstrate the alpha rhythms of the human brain, which oscillate at a frequency of eight to thirteen cycles per second.

Around the same time, osteopath William G. Sutherland was practicing and teaching in Mankato, Minnesota. In 1899, while a student at the American School of Osteopathy, he viewed a disarticulated skull which belonged to Andrew Taylor Still, the founder of Osteopathy. The beveled articular surfaces, relative to the greater wings of the sphenoid and the squamous portions of the temporal bone, were especially intriguing. Suddenly, " . . . like a blinding flash of light came the thought: beveled like the gills of a fish and indicating articular mobility for a respiratory mechanism." As he searched for a reference through countless volumes of anatomy and physiology, he could find no hint of this concept. He tried to put the thought out of his mind, wanting to be neither contrary nor outspoken. But over the next few years the thought kept creeping back in. His eventual experiments strengthened his conviction. Holding that no design of anatomy is without purpose, and in a spirit similar to the great homeopathic provings, Sutherland quietly began a series of bizarre investigations. After careful study of the cranial articulations and relationships, he rigged a series of ingenious leather devices designed to restrain the bones of his cranium and strapped them onto his head. Here his wife recalls his account of an early breakthrough experiment:

> With no accurate understanding of the use to which they would be put, I helped in lacing together two catcher's mitts, and observed as a buckle was attached to one, and an adjustable strap to the other. Will then rested his head upon the laced mitts to test their contour, which was similar to the V-shape headrest of a dental chair.
>
> "I wonder what Will will be doing if not busy with a patient?" That was my thought each time I turned officeward. One day upon arriving there I learned with startling abruptness that the "doing" had been done.
>
> His color was unnatural, his appearance feverish, and his manner disturbingly preoccupied... He explained that the experiment to compress the fourth ventricle had just had its initial tryout. He told of lying down, his head in the V-shape headrest; of imposing compression by gradual tension of buckle and strap. He described the sensations he had experienced as he approached near-unconsciousness. And that although weakened he had succeeded in releasing the leverage strap. "A sensation of warmth followed," he explained. "And also a remarkable movement of fluid, up and down the spinal column, throughout the ventricles, and surrounding the brain." His physical experience he summed up in one word: "Fantastic!"
>
> "Believe it or not, there also was a movement of my sacrum! What are we getting into? Is there no end to this?"

Thus Sutherland serendipitously discovered the reciprocal tension relationship of the cranium and sacrum. He continued his study for 55 years, keeping his work mostly to himself for the first thirty. In 1932 he first presented his concepts to the American Osteopathic Association, itself an outcast group in the world of science, and was not well received. By this time, having devoted three decades to single-minded study of every possible aspect of the cranium, its bones and articulations, its membranes, and its function in relationship to the rest of the body, he was confident of his observations. He returned undaunted to his clinic in Mankato, Minnesota, and continued to conduct re-

Figure 22: William
Sutherland D.O.

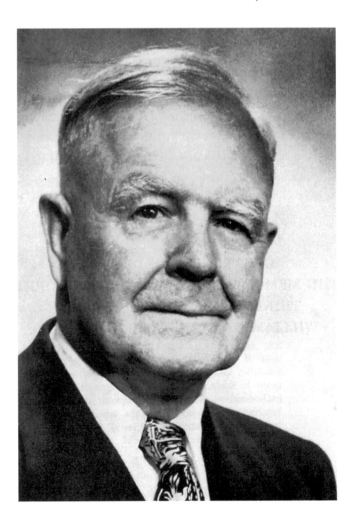

search and teach for another 25 years. William Sutherland died in 1954, barely recognized but not in the least bitter. A self-motivated man, his satisfaction in life came from his devotion to clinical practice, where his principles served him unfailingly.

Holding that force begets resistance, Sutherland was fond of telling the story of the North Wind and the Sun, who made a wager that each could remove a man's coat. The infamous North Wind had first try, and with all his substantial might concentrated his breath singularly on the poor man. But the harder he blew, the tighter the man pulled his coat around his body. Finally he gave up, and the Sun had his turn. He came out smiling, patient and confident, paying no particular mind to the man but gently radiating warmth over all the earth. In a manner of minutes, the man took off his coat. This story reveals Dr. Sutherland's conviction that the autonomic system is a sensible and willful entity, demonstrating what chiropractic calls "innate intelligence." His fundamental principle: "To allow the physiological function within to manifest its unerring potency, rather than the application of blind force from without."

By the time of Sutherland's death, cranial manipulation had gained a foothold among certain osteopaths and chiropractors. But the general scientific community to this day scoffs, if it bothers to respond at all, at the concept of cranial articular mobility and a cranial respiratory mechanism. It is presently not considered respectable to study the activity of the brain without measuring instruments. This presents a bit of a problem, because to disturb the meninges by the introduction of needles, instrumentation, etc., tends to alter the hydrodynamics of the system (the "Heisenberg dilemma"). Also, because the cranial vault expands to maintain pressure homeostasis in the CSF system, there is no measurable fluctuation of pressure. Sutherland himself did not fret over these problems, trusting the reliable sensitivity of his own nervous system as a clinical and research instrument. In recent years, there has been successful objective measurement of rhythmic cranial fluctuation and cranial articular mobility (see Upledger's *Craniosacral Therapy,* appendices). It is likely that the craniosacral concept will eventually gain wide recognition.

Sutherland's concept of craniosacral function, including cranial bone motion, cerebrospinal fluid fluctuation, and meningeal reciprocal tension, seems to hold true to his insight in its virtual entirety. Details have been elaborated and a few points clarified, but today, after almost a hundred years of research and clinical practice, the physiology seems true to his original vision. Of course, what interests us is the clinical application. The data is largely subjective, frequently anecdotal, and basically encouraging.

There has been since Sutherland a lineage of great cranial osteopaths (craniopaths) in the U.S. and Europe who made significant conceptual and clinical contributions to the field. For the most part, they have endeavored to keep the cranial concept strictly within the osteopathic domain, refusing to teach cranial techniques to chiropractors much as some chiropractors today seek to withhold certain practices from physical therapists.

The Craniosacral Concept in Chiropractic

In 1936, Nephi Cottam, D.C., published *The Story of Craniopathy,* in which he discussed his clinical research into cranial adjusting dating back to the 1920s. Cottam's admonition was "to spread—spread—spread. Give more space. Don't 'jam.' Spread apart within the vault." James R. Alberts, D.C., also advocated the treatment of the cranium by spreading the sutures. This is an excellent idea.

Besides tractioning open the cranial joints, it exercises sutural proprioceptors that reflect into the fluid pressure system.

In addition to spreading the sutures, it is valuable to work the superficial cranial muscles and proprioceptors. When working these structures it might be appropriate to drop in to a stronger, but not brute, degree of pressure in comparison to the delicate attitude that is appropriate in approaching the intracranial milieu.

In 1959, James Alberts published Alberts' *Cerebral Meningeal Stress Syndrome: A Primary Release of the Central Nervous System Related to Shock and Stress*. In his book and teachings, Dr. Alberts discussed the relationship between the cranium, meningeal tension, and emotional stress. Alberts also developed a neurologic model of cranial function that regards the neurologic organization of fault patterns and serves as a foundation for much of the Applied Kinesiology cranial concept.

Leo L. Spears, D.C., founder of the original chiropractic hospital—the 800-bed Spears Chiropractic Sanitarium in Denver, Colorado—developed a system he called Cranial Remolding in which cranial distortion was analyzed according to quadrants and without regard to the sutures, and correction delivered by applying rhythmic intermittent pressure to the skull of a seated patient. Spears emphasized the events of improper natal delivery as the causative factor in cranial problems and took a special interest in the application of "cranial re-shaping" in cases of cerebral palsy.

A principal chiropractic proponent of technique based on full consideration of the craniosacral system has been M.B. DeJarnette, D.C. His Sacro-Occipital Technic (SOT) is a unique and imaginative utilization of the physiologic model first developed by Sutherland, who had been teaching in Minnesota for a generation by the time of DeJarnette's graduation from Palmer College. There is evidence that a young DeJarnette visited Sutherland's school. Dr. DeJarnette developed a whole-body approach with an appreciation of reciprocal tension and from a chiropractic vantage. His pelvic block technique remains an original and significant innovation in core system therapeutics. Dr. DeJarnette also held to the unity of structure and function, and of visceral and somatic relationships. He developed an inspired clinical concept utilizing visual and palpatory analysis, neuroreflex stimulation, and visceral manipulation (the powerful "Bloodless Surgery") called "Chiropractic Manipulative Reflex Techniques" (CMRT), which he coupled with a profound structural technique to increase neurologic and biomechanical efficiency.

Unfortunately, as has so often occurred in chiropractic, in communicating his ideas to the world Dr. DeJarnette found a limited audience. The world at large simply was not listening. Also, DeJarnette chose to present his concepts in a series of annual "yearbooks" that mirrored the doctor's folksy and didactic approach and featured a spontaneous workshop format which lacked consistency of presentation from issue to issue, was without an index, and which featured an unsophisticated illustration technique that does no justice to the profundity of his concept. The physiological breadth of DeJarnette's technique is astounding, encompassing biomechanical, craniosacral, nutritional and chemical, neuromuscular and visceral, neurologic and psychosomatic aspects of function.

SOT cranial technique was, for many chiropractors, our first exposure to the craniosacral concept. DeJarnette maintained a somewhat proprietary attitude towards cranial technique, warning that the cranium is a vulnerable mechanism that can be the cause of iatrogenic malfunction, and therefore claimed suzerainty over the teaching and clinical use of the concept. He adopted a view of sutural (bony) fixation as a therapeutic focus in treatment and utilized exteroceptive palpation, visual observation, and structural and neurologic indicators as clues in analysis. The SOT cranial treatment procedures tend to be a bit more heavy-handed than those presented here, probably the reason for DeJarnette's warning.

A further proponent of cranial treatment in chiropractic has been George Goodheart, D.C., the father of Applied Kinesiology (AK). Dr. Goodheart expanded considerably on the chiropractic and SOT basis. AK is rooted firmly in chiropractic but is uniquely original. With his natural curiosity perhaps his greatest strength, Dr. Goodheart developed in AK an intuitive basis for examination procedures that has almost universal application. The body of AK defines a great deal of the operating system of the adapting human organism. It is "simply profound and profoundly simple."

In exploring the neurocranial function, Goodheart established that there are 14 basic "cranial faults," which correlate directly with specific patterns of breathing, and in fact seem to present cranial bone motility as a secondary effect of pneumatic respiration. This does not account for the fact that the cranial respiratory pattern can be palpated even while the subject is holding his breath. The motion of the craniosacral rhythm is inherent to the central nervous system. This is the basis for Sutherland's labeling of the craniosacral rhythm as the "primary respiratory mechanism" which, he theorized, provides the underlying stimulus for pneumatic respiration through its rhythmic effect on the pontine respiratory center beneath the floor of the fourth ventricle.

The AK approach to cranial technique utilizes neurologic muscle indicators in conjunction with specific breathing activity to determine the need for correction of cranial bone fixation and breathing fixation patterns. It also, in various ways, relates craniosacral mechanisms and relationships to total body organization (physiology). The approach presented here varies from AK in that we will palpate the fluid pressure and tension pattern directly as an indicator of the patient's dynamic state. This parallels Selye's principle of stress as an overall, nonspecific physiologic response in addition to all of the specific responses. "Anything can cause anything" in the hydraulic membrane system; therefore, while the superficial osseous pattern is observed and noted, it is not too seriously analyzed. It is a handle on the dynamic state, most useful simply as a point of departure for change. In this spirit, there will be times when we won't attempt to directly "fix" anything, but will endeavor instead to communicate satisfactorily, proprioceptively and interoceptively, in assisting our patient to subtly, simply, and fundamentally change herself. If, however, our efforts fail to clear the indicators demonstrated by screen and panel, AK testing, or any other criteria, the standard procedures should be considered.

There is no intention here to slight chiropractic, but rather to suggest a conceptual framework, "from the inside out," that explains, complements, and refines the chiropractic concept without substantially interfering with it. There may, of course, be specific things about a patient that can, should, and must be "fixed" by direct and forceful interaction. This is the very basis of the relationship with our patient, not something to be taken fancifully. But like the famous parable of the wind and the sun, there are certain things, fundamental things, that cannot be changed in this way. So we add to our "bag of tricks," and sometimes the tricks themselves transform us.

In recent years, valuable chiropractic research into craniosacral physiology has been conducted by Lowell Ward, D.C. Comprehending that "the spine is a singular synchronous functional unit," he developed in Spinal Column Stressology a means of objectifying meningeal distortion and the psychoemotional states that accompany it, as well as the relationship of spinal patterns to adaptation.

Mark Pick, D.C., of Los Angeles, California, has also made a substantial contribution to the cranial field in chiropractic. Well known as an anatomist, his experimental approach to the anatomy and physiology of the craniosacral system, via SOT, is legendary in chiropractic.

John Upledger

I learned craniosacral work from John Upledger, D.O., F.A.A.O., of Palm Beach, Florida, author of the definitive texts *Craniosacral Therapy, Volumes 1 & 2* (Eastland Press, Chicago, 1983 and Eastland Press, Seattle, 1987) and widely regarded as the authority in the field. Upledger impressed me from the start with his lack of pretension, his depth of understanding, his clinical acumen, and his willingness to share what he knows without demanding anything in return. He has his head in the clouds, but his feet are firmly planted in earth.

Upledger began as an osteopathic general practitioner, utilizing a pharmaceutical and surgical protocol. While assisting on a neurosurgery, he drew criticism for his inability to hold the dura steady to the satisfaction of the surgeon. No matter how he tried, the dura crawled with a life of its own and would not submit to control. This began an inquiry that led through human and simian dissections and thousands of hours of clinical research and interdisciplinary rigor to the dynamic anatomic and functional concept known as Craniosacral Therapy (CST).

Upledger led an interdisciplinary team of researchers at the University of Michigan in the 1970s that verified and documented the phenomenon of cranial respiratory motion in the body. He also pioneered a clinical approach to autistic children with a great measure of success. He recounts the irony of achieving a major breakthrough with a child, only to find that the previously predictable child was now being perceived by the institutional staff as troublesome and therefore incurring punishment.

The Upledger approach to the craniosacral system is rooted in osteopathy but is at the same time distinctly original. His emphasis on human concerns stands as an obvious but often overlooked reminder of what is really going on here. For Upledger, the human heart is at the core of the human brain.

Stress Storage in the Membrane System

*I*t's well known that mental and emotional issues usually involve somatic tension. It has been observed clinically that body tension often has mental and emotional implications. Sometimes in releasing somatic tension patterns a patient will encounter significant emotion that may (or may not) be associated with memories of past experience. Often these memories are painful, and he may be surprised by them, indicating that the memories have until now been blocked from active recall. In these cases the patient may come to the realization that his body symptom is somehow related to the suppression of the experience and the feelings associated with it. The observation of these phenomena raises questions as to the nature of stress storage in the body.

We commonly use the term "stress" to imply "distress," but "stress" really implies any demand for processing or adaptation on the part of the organism, including demands which we may find enjoyable. Because "stress" refers to the non-specific response on the part of the body in its mobilization to action, even pleasure can be perceived as distress by the organism if it presents a significant demand for autonomic response at the wrong time (the "Nelson Rockefeller Syndrome"). In general, only "distress" will be stored by a body, signifying that the organism was unsuccessful in satisfactorily processing or adapting to a challenge. This stress is therefore stored in the tissues as potential energy which may be experienced and palpated as tissue tension and its effects.

The Mechanism of Stress Storage in the Membrane Structure

Stress may be stored in the body for at least two reasons. First, we are capable of maintaining neurologic reconfigurations adopted in response to past physiologic malfunction. Second, there may be a similar mechanism which represents psychoemotional "unfinished business." Both phenomena often demonstrate short-term advantages and long-term disadvantages. The neurology of adaptation is a considerable subject and goes beyond our topic. We will consider the tensile aspects here, with neurologic function always in mind.

Somatic expression of feelings occurs naturally and spontaneously by virtue of the fact that the body tissues are pervaded by the nervous system. The membrane-musculoskeletal system is especially abundant with innervation, and its configurations are direct representations of brain-function configurations. We all recognize the facial expressions and body habitus of joy, sadness, anger, and other feelings. The inability to thoroughly and satisfactorily process a stress may be associated with these neurologic body patterns on a long-term basis. This often involves feelings with which the person is unable to come to terms or fully accept. The person may consciously be unaware of the conflict, and may even believe that the problem is satisfactorily resolved, but the body is less capable of self-deception and may hold the unresolved situation in storage as a tissue pattern that represents the position in which the body was configured and the somatoemotional expression at the time of the trauma. Traumas may routinely be physical in origin, such as accidents and medical procedures, and they may be associated with feelings of pain, shock, or resentment. They may also derive from the unacceptable behavior of other individuals toward the subject, or from the subject's unacceptance of his own behavior. The understanding of these phenomena requires a sincere respect for "body wisdom," which leads us to ask "why?" before we make our diagnostic and therapeutic impressions. The body does what it does deliberately and intelligently as the consequence of being presented with options of behavior, none of which may be totally advantageous. It will usually choose the most advantageous and viable option given the limitations of the situation and the will of the person.

The "stress dilemma" may be stated as an incompatibility between the will to function and a limited ability to provide that function. The autonomic system is a slave to our will, subjugating itself to the will to the best of its ability for as long as it can. In other words, the nervous system when confronted by a challenge reorganizes itself to "get the job done." At the same time, unresolved conflicts remain unresolved, and are in effect put on the back burner where they may stew and possibly burn.

Holding and Breakdown Patterns

One aspect of stress storage in the body manifests as patterns of tension in the reciprocal-tension membrane system. This patterning represents the interface between the physical and psychoemotional aspects of the self. It is not the membrane tissue itself, but the configuration of the membrane system that is significant here. A pattern is energetic (behavioral) in nature; thus we can use the tension pattern to assess the energetic status of our patient. The tension patterns are of two natures:

Holding patterns represent a configuration of the tissue/membrane system in expression of chronic psycho-emotional states. We are all familiar with the hunched-over habitus of poor self-esteem, or the puffed-up chest of pride. These represent more obvious examples of body habitus. The membrane system is also capable of subtle chronic patterning by which it holds specific emotional traumas which do not read in such an obvious manner. Sometimes the only way to interpret such patterns is through hindsight after they are released with the accompaniment of memories and/or emotion. Patterns may also be released without either memories or emotion, in which case it may be impossible to ascertain their origin. Tissue holding patterns represent "brain" holding patterns.

Another type of holding pattern represents a long-term neurologic adaptation to a chronic behavioral tendency. Typical of this type of holding pattern is the subluxation-fixation of the sixth thoracic vertebra in a person with a chronic glucose metabolism problem and a persistent sweet tooth. This represents a classic stress dilemma. The subluxation is autonomically deliberate.

Breakdown patterns represent the effects of physical trauma and micro-trauma which result from injuries, disease processes, and chronic body use patterns. A common tendency of breakdown patterns involves the influence of gravity on body structures, possibly in conjunction with the effects of traumatic injury.

As previously mentioned, when confronted with the will to function and a limited ability to provide that function, we are capable of neurologic reconfiguring as a means of getting by. The nervous system also has the uncanny ability to learn to recognize any configuration in which it must function as the normal state. It may therefore carry old adaptive patterns which no longer serve it efficiently and instead represent an ongoing burden to the system. The AK reactive muscle pattern is an example of this and may be seen as both a breakdown pattern (demand) and a physiologic holding pattern (response) adopted intentionally. These cases may respond quite well to standard therapeutic procedures and exercise.

Holding and breakdown patterns may be intimately related, as in the case of an injury which is accompanied by fear, resentment, or anger and also involves a long recuperative period which results in financial burden; another example would be a person who develops osteoarthritis or disc herniation from years of sitting at a desk job which she hates. Post-surgical scars also present a challenging example of combined influences. The two pattern types may exist relatively independent of one another; however, it is advantageous to consider that the reason the patient acquired the symptom and the reason that he or she is retaining the symptom may be two separate issues. It is also important to consider that a breakdown pattern may encounter a previously existing breakdown pattern (for example, deep cicatrix) which may complicate the patient's recovery to a significant degree.

The adaptive disadvantage common to both holding and breakdown patterns is that they require so much autonomic energy to maintain, especially considering the cost of the behavior patterns which may spring from them. This dramatically reduces the adaptive reserve available to the organism.

Holding and breakdown membrane patterns exhibit reciprocal influence with somatic pressure gradients in the various body compartments. Stanley Keleman, in his book *Emotional Anatomy,* offers some insights into pressure gradients in illustrated form. Other pressure gradients, such as swollen or hypertrophied viscera, inflammations, etc., will also find expression in the reciprocal-tension membrane system. This subject expands far beyond our present discussion.

Traumatically Induced Stress Vectors

Physical traumas are characterized by the body's absorption of an impact vector, and the force of collision can in some cases represent substantial kinetic energy. The body may dissipate some of the energy through motion (for example, by falling or being thrown) and may dissipate some as heat (as in inflammation) and it may also store some of the force as potential energy. The latter seems especially likely in the case of damaging trauma that induces the victim to improvise function while in the recuperative state (a classic stress dilemma), or injury accompanied by severe pain or emotional or financial impact. The body assigns the vector potential to a "second priority" holding pattern in the membrane system and lays a neurologic "patch cord" around it so that the organism may function, free to attend to the immediate agenda. Now, in a sense, it is sealed in membrane, an "energy cyst," as Upledger calls it. In ten days or two weeks it may be integrated into the framework of the normal working model of the self and may remain "invisible" but unresolved for years to come, heard but not seen.

Stress Patterns in the Craniosacral Membrane

The central nervous system is the structural and functional axis of the body. All tension patterns in the somatic structure are capable of manifestation in the core membrane through reciprocal tension and neurologic holding patterns. This model is consistent with ancient concepts of yoga which traditionally view stress as torsion on the spinal cord. Many meditation techniques and the postures of hatha yoga address this phenomenon directly. In your therapeutic approach, consider the torsion on the dura in relationship to any other details you perceive in your patient.

Fixations

Fixation is the condition of being held in a fixed position. Both hard and soft tissue fixations often involve the deposition of "cheap-grade" fibrous adhesions which hold the tissue in one place or within a limited phase of its potential range of motion on a long-term basis. This has obvious bearing on mobility, posture, and comfort. It also can restrict motility and subsequently vitality. Adhesions are deposited in the body by the transformation of latent fibrinogen into fiber, which occurs secondary to swelling, inflammation, scarring, immobility, and any other state characterized by stasis of membrane motion and/or fluid flow. Fixations are the representation of old business, like scars but differing from cicatrix in several ways.

As is often the case in adaptive behavior, due to the inherent immediacy the survival dilemma, our body may produce an effect that has short-term advantages and long-term disadvantages. This is typical of many adhesive fixations. But there may sometimes be deliberate cause for the deposition of fiber. Chronic holding patterns require energy to hold the pattern, and adhesions may serve the body well in this function while freeing up the autonomic focus for more immediate concerns. This may be the case in our above example of the sixth thoracic fixation-subluxation. Thus in breaking somatic fixation patterns, it may be important to address the behavior patterns of the individual as well, in order to avoid robbing the patient of her intentional and much-needed adaptation.

Applied Kinesiology uses the term "fixation" to describe a pattern of bilateral muscle failure indicative of postural maladaptation. This type of fixation represents a physiologic holding pattern in response to a weight-bearing break-down demand.

There are bony fixations as well. Bony (hard) fixations, if of a short dura-tion, may exhibit little or no fibrous deposition. They occur when the joint is allowed by the musculomembrane tension system to separate, either trauma-tically or microtraumatically, and the bones are allowed to shift in relationship to one another. Then the joint tension is reestablished and the joint is pulled taut in the aberrant relationship. Bony fixations are capable of fixating the membrane system in abnormal tension patterns.

Thrusting adjustments are contraindicated for cranial fixations. Hard fix-ations elsewhere in the body can respond quite well to thrusting adjustment techniques; however, if they return it may be advantageous to consider the soft-tissue tension system, which represents a system of cables that stabilize the joints. Imagine a kink in a chain. As long as the tension on the chain is main-tained, it will not be easy to remove the kink. But if the tensity is relaxed, the kink can be unwound and the tension can then be safely reintroduced.

The deeper a fixation in the body, the more widespread is its influence in restricting both mobility and motility throughout the organism. Because the craniosacral system represents the body's core membrane, and also because it is the nervous system and constitutes the main communication and coordi-nating system, adhesive fixations within it may result in myriad complaints and malfunctions.

Fixation is also a term with psychological implications. In classical Freudian terms, it refers to the arrest of development at one phase in the natural se-quence of maturation which results in "neurotic" behavior, characterized by vulnerability, an inappropriate response to situations and relationships, and a failure to find satisfaction in day-to-day life. Freud was especially interested in fixations acquired during early stages of psychosexual development, but oth-ers have broadened the concept to recognize any traumatic experience as a po-tential source of fixation. The earlier the maladjustment, the deeper the fixation and the more likely is one to be "fixated as a permanent disorder" (Freud). The correlation between psychological and physical fixation is striking, both con-ceptually and clinically. Not all body patterns have emotional roots, but vir-tually all emotional problems find somatic expression.

Releasing Stress Patterns

As the core membrane, the craniosacral system offers us therapeutic access to subtle membrane patterns which represent the storage of chronic stress, and which through reciprocal tension may transfer these tensions to distal and seemingly unrelated structures, leading to "idiopathic" symptomatology. It becomes apparent that in assisting the patient in freeing himself from the bonds of such patterns, we may at times encounter situations which are "psychological" in nature. It may be appropriate to refer such a patient for counseling. It is also appropriate to learn to recognize the unity of mind and body and to therefore develop our skills in dealing with these matters as they arise. Sometimes in the process of recall and release, old and negative behavior patterns which are predicated on past traumas can terrify the patient initially and seem less terrifying in hindsight. The patient, healed of the physical manifestation, may still require referral for counseling. Each doctor chooses her level of involvement with her patients and develops specific skills. Because the boundaries are by and large synthetic ones, it would be a shame to deny our patients the reality of mind-body unity and therefore the opportunity to further integrate their function.

Other mechanisms of stress storage and interactions between stress configurations, including adaptive neurologic patterning and reconfiguration, are not discussed here.

Reciprocal Tension

*E*ach somatic structure is invested with a semipermeable connective tissue envelope: myofascia, periosteum, epineurium, perineurium, endoneurium, the meninges, tunica adventitia, organ capsule, pleurae, pericardium, etc. In addition, there are numerous fascial sheaths which form body compartments or serve as a suspensory matrix for the viscerae, including the diaphragm, peritoneum, mesentery, omentum, etc. Ligaments also qualify as connective tissue membrane. These membranes blend microscopically with one another and with the tissue stroma, and anchor strategically to one another and to bones. These reciprocal connections form the basis of tension relationships that are capable of transmitting vector forces to distal regions. This mechanism moves our body, and it may also hinder it from motion.

In other words, every tension vector has two ends. If you tug on your sleeve, you can feel the pull on your shoulder. Notice that if you pull on the front of your shirt, you can feel it in both shoulders, on the sides of your ribs, above and below, etc. This is reciprocal tension.

In the craniosacral system, there are classically two reciprocal tension membranes (RTM), cranial and spinal, separated by the firm attachment of the dura to the foramen magnum. The cranial RTM includes the intracranial membranes considered as a unified structure: falx cerebri, falx cerebelli, and tentorium cerebellum, which act around the fulcrum of the straight sinus to exert an influence on the cranial bones. When you hold the head, feel for this membrane tension and its expression of the intracranial fluid pressure. The spinal RTM is the semi-freely gliding dural tube from the foramen magnum to the attachment of the filum terminale externum at the first coccygeal segment.

In reality, there is really one functional reciprocal tension membrane, a collagen organ which includes not only the intracranial and meningeal aspects of the craniosacral membrane, but virtually all of the membranes and even the stroma of the body in conjunction with the levering effect of bones and the tension influence of various fluid pressure gradients. The total picture can be complex and difficult to analyze. Fortunately, it can with some practice be palpated directly.

To develop an awareness of reciprocal tension in the body is to open up an intuitive avenue of perception that allows us to understand the relationship between distal structures. A dislocated acromioclavicular joint, for example, can create a tension that is transmitted through the fascia of the back to the lumbosacral area, creating a symptom of low back pain and vulnerability. In such a case, there is no therapeutic modality that can be applied successfully to the back to relieve the symptom, but the ability to directly feel the reciprocal tension relationship can attract attention to the cause of the problem in the shoulder. This same principle can be applied to spinal or cranial tensions, organ or fascial adhesions, or any other structural limitation that refers its effects to distal structures.

An appreciation of restrictions in the craniosacral system will orient you to the deepest structural reality. From this vantage you can learn to perceive tension relationships from the inside out to the fascia and organs. In addition, you can learn to palpate reciprocal tension from the superficial structures to the deep.

Practice

This exercise requires three people. A and B hold the corners of a rectangle of plastic wrap and pull the wrap taut. Their eyes are closed. The third person C pokes the cloth gently in various places, first with one finger and then adding a second poke with another finger while the two holding the membrane observe by feel the location of the interference. It will be quite easy. Experiment with how subtle an interference can be palpated.

Now C closes her eyes. A and B hold the membrane taut using their thumb and middle finger, and one of them uses a free finger to create with a pull, various types of subtle tension vectors. C palpates the surface of the membrane with a flat hand while making proprioceptive observations about the nature of the tension pattern. Now add multiple pulls.

The Nature of Palpation

Human physiology exists perpetually in the fluid state; that is, it fluxes constantly as it processes, moves, and copes. Palpation offers us a means by which we can appreciate physiology in the fluid state, a means that is "totally subjective and completely reliable" (Upledger).

Passive and Active Palpation: The Fluid Nature of Rhythm

Active palpation utilizes the application of digital pressure (pacinian corpuscles) or movement to assess parameters such as range of motion, pain sensitivity, shape, consistency, muscle tension, etc., and may induce a response or movement in the subject.

Passive palpation utilizes minimal pressure and movement so that the physiologic motion of the whole organism can be appreciated in a relatively undisturbed state. In developing appreciation of the craniosacral rhythm and other subtle motions of the organism, passive palpation is the choice. Because we are perceiving wave motion through a liquid medium it is best to avoid setting any extraneous waves into motion with our palpation. Active palpation used inappropriately may also induce a defensive tension response in the neuromusculature of the subject, and this tension will tend to interfere with the tissue's ability to transmit the inherent wave activity accurately. Lastly, motion on the part of the palpator involves motor activity of the palpating hand and competes with the perception of the sensory tracts.

Palpating The Continuum: Gross to Subtle

The body represents a spectrum of tissue density from gross to subtle. Hard tissue, soft tissue, membrane tension patterns, fluid wave patterns, and subtle energy can all be palpated. The craniosacral rhythm represents a unifying wave pattern through the spectrum of densities. The ability to grasp the continuum of this spectrum at once, as it exists, offers us the opportunity to appreciate the patient in a way not available by any other means.

Table 1: The Spectrum of Densities	
Gross	**Subtle**
bone	
soft tissue	
membrane tension	
fluid wave patterns	

Note: "Energy" in humans refers to behavior (activity) and to the ability (potential) to behave. Behavior may be willful, "subconscious," or autonomic. Autonomic energy (activity) tends to move in patterns (rhythm). Organization of activity is the basis of good function, the "secret" of good health.

Proprioceptive and Tactile Palpation

There are two primary conscious sensory pathways in the CNS. The **spinothalamic** tract transmits **exteroceptive** sensations which arise from stimuli outside the self. These include pain, temperature, and objective touch. The spinothalamic fibers cross in the cord and ascend to the thalamus. This tract is also responsible for viscerosomatic sensations and plays a role in the "gating" mechanism of pain limitation.

The **dorsal column-lemniscal** pathway carries conscious **proprioceptive** sensations which arise within the body, including sense of position of the musculoskeletal components at rest, kinesthetic sense of the body in motion, and vibratory sensation (pattern organization of touch). It also has tactile discrimination fibers which define the subjective tactile sense, including that of texture and pressure. This pathway ascends in the dorsal columns of the cord and crosses in the medulla oblongata just before synapsing at the nuclei cuneatus and gracilis. It then proceeds as the medial lemniscus to the thalamus. **Interoception** refers to the autonomic ascending pathways.

There is a third spinocerebellar pathway for unconscious proprioception, which is in intimate communication with the conscious sense. The two pathways of conscious perception provide the basis of the bipalpatory concept.

Figure 23: *Dorsal column-lemniscal pathway (left) spinothalamic tract (right)*

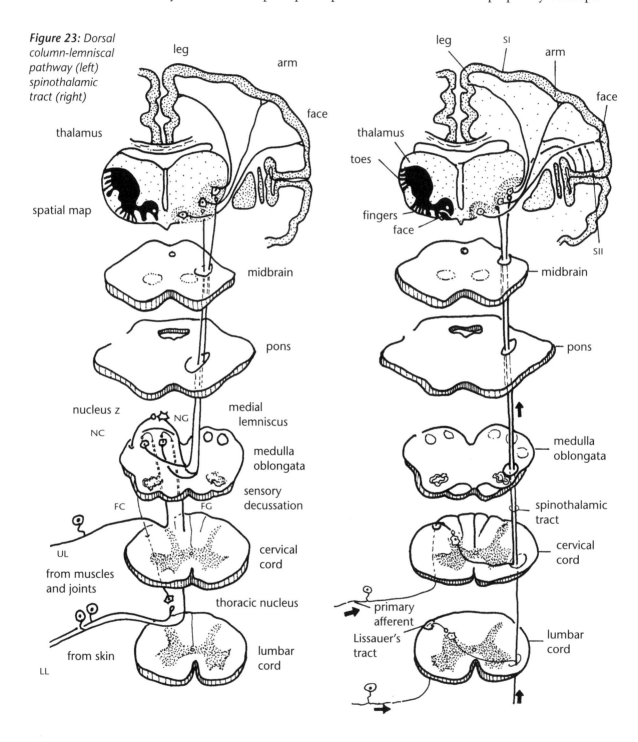

leg
arm
face
thalamus
spatial map
midbrain
pons
nucleus z
NG
NC
medial lemniscus
medulla oblongata
sensory decussation
FC
FG
cervical cord
UL
from muscles and joints
thoracic nucleus
from skin
LL
lumbar cord

leg
SI
arm
face
thalamus
toes
fingers
face
SII
midbrain
pons
medulla oblongata
spinothalamic tract
cervical cord
primary afferent
Lissauer's tract
lumbar cord

Table 2: Conscious Sensory Routes

Tracts	
Spinothalamic	Dorsal column-lemniscal
exteroception	conscious proprioception
objective touch (stereognosis)	subjective touch (and fine gradation)
pain (nociception)	body position at rest
thermal	kinesthetic sense
viscerosomatic	vibratory (pattern of pressure and touch)
poor spatial definition	spatially specific (homunculus)
slow (1-15 mps)	fast (30-75 mps)

The active palpating hand utilizes motor activity (movement and pressure) and sensory activity (tactile discrimination) to discriminate between its activity and that of the subject, as perceived at the boundary between palpator and subject. It is a probe, and its nature is to "delve into" tissue and discover information. Objective tactile discrimination is exteroceptive and occurs at the dermal and epidermal level (body surface) with the activation of tactile skin receptors.

The Vibratory Sense

The vibratory sense perceives organization in biphasic touch activity (rhythm). The rhythm can be binary (digital) or wave-form (analog) and may be easily organized or may seem random. Vibratory sensation ascends with the proprioceptive tracts.

The Blended Hand

The passive palpating hand "blends" with the subject, bypassing the tactile receptors. When learning to palpate proprioceptively, it is useful to avoid focusing on the hands at first. Use the proprioceptive mechanism of your wrists, forearms, elbows, and arms as your main sensory instrument. From this vantage the hand proprioceptors are also readily available, especially in the interossei and opponens muscles.

It is the proprioceptive tracts that allow us to know our own body position in the dark. Most of us regard this as a sensitive and absolutely reliable system. The blended hand is by its quiet nature fully sensory, and as it is also fluid it rides with the wave pattern of that with which it is blended. In proprioceptive palpation, discriminate between one part of yourself (distal forearm/wrist, elbow) and another (proximal forearm/elbow) as a means of understanding the milieu of your subject. The dorsal columns provide us with "an instantaneous body image at the level of the somatic sensory cortex" (Fitzgerald). The development of this conscious and inherent imaging phenomenon, in conjunction with the blended hand, allows us to perceive our patient in a subjective physiologic state. The human nervous system is as complex and sensitive a sensory device as has ever been devised "by God or Man." There are myriad implications to the old adage "Know yourself" in this practice.

Subjectivity in Palpation

The nervous system is a specialized communication system. Palpation is a purely subjective skill that allows us to communicate with the nervous system itelf. The willfulness of the human central nervous system is well documented. As the experience of life, conscious and autonomic, is largely subjective it seems appropriate that this appreciation be developed. Passive palpation is listening and requires presence. Perhaps the less one says about what he palpates, the better we can trust that person's palpatory efficacy. The idea is not to give the patient advice, but to listen as the patient expresses herself, something she does inherently every moment of her life. In chiropractic we call this innate intelligence.

Training the Senses

For the purpose of training ourselves to utilize proprioceptive palpation, the exercises below will discourage the use of active palpation. The clinical practitioner of course takes appropriate advantage of both active and passive palpation, and with the acquisition of skill learns to appreciate both sensory tracts simultaneously with the motor function.

The Sensory Basis of Motor Function: The Long Loop

Inherent to the motor function is the concept of intent. Intentional use of the body derives neurologically from the motor cortex and beyond that from a nebulous locale, the place in us where thought originates. Afferent impulses to the motorneurons also originate from the sensory tracts as either cord reflex or **"long loop"** reflex via the dorsal column-lemniscal pathway to the sensorimotor cortex. In this way intentional motor activity relies on feedback mechanisms from that which we feel. The **long loop** pathway involves a conscious sensory tract and a conscious motor tract. (It also plays a major role in muscle testing.) Train your focus on the long loop for palpation. The implication, of course, is that in delivering care to your patient, the motor function actively relies on the proprioceptive reality of the patient's physiologic state, and this allows a more direct communication with the patient.

Selective Focus

The craniosacral, vascular, and breathing rhythms can all be palpated from any vantage. Train yourself to bring your attention to any one aspect of this phenomenon and then "wipe clean" your sentient field and refocus on another aspect. Thus from any listening station you can perceive first the vascular pulsations, then the breathing rhythm, and then the craniosacral rhythm, and switch back and forth among them at will. Selective focus also allows you to alternate between exteroceptive and proprioceptive sensory circuits as you palpate.

Palpation of Poise

Poise is the resting attitude of the organism. Poise is physical (body habitus), mental (thought), and emotional (feeling). Structural poise is the way the body holds itself at rest (in neutral), including all of the joint relationships, muscle tension patterns, etc. Poise cannot be described, predicted, or quantified. Aspects of poise can be measured but are in all cases inefficient in relating the essence of its nature. Poise can be palpated proprioceptively as a spontaneous impression. Let it in. Focusing your attention on poise enables you to "lock in" to the tension pattern of your patient so that you can interact with it.

Practice: Proprioceptive Perception

Two partners.

Partner A: Hold your hands out, palms up.

Partner B: Your hands rest on your partner's hands. Relax your hands and keep your touch light.

A: Rotate your hands gently to approximate the Cranial Respiratory Impulse. See how subtle a motion you can create.

B: Close your eyes and feel the motion in your forearms and elbows. See how subtle a motion you can perceive.

Practice: Membrane Tension

Three partners. These short and simple exercises demonstrate the straightforward concept of palpating membrane tension. It can be just about this easy to feel distal tension in the body. These same exercises are also included in the chapter on reciprocal tension.

1. A and B: Hold the corners of a sheet of plastic wrap and pull it taut. Each partner can slightly exaggerate the pull on one corner for a moment to demonstrate reciprocal tension.

C: Poke the "membrane" gently with your finger from above and below. See how subtle an interference you can create.

A and B: With your eyes closed, identify the location of the finger. See how subtle an interference you can identify.

C: Now poke your finger at an angle to introduce a vector component.

2. A and B: Same as above.

C: Hold your open hand to the surface of the membrane.

A and B: Create reciprocal tension from the corners of the membrane. Add additional vectors with a free finger while C identifies the source of the interference.

Practice: Palpation of Poise and Rhythms on Self

Sit comfortably and raise your arms. Bend your elbows and place your hands gently on your head with your fingers comfortably spread. Your wrists are suspended like slings from your elbows. With your touch as light as possible, alight on the skull like water spiders on surface tension. Your thumbs are under your occipital base and your fifth fingers grace the sides of your frontal. Rest at the interface of your scalp and the atmosphere, and then settle in to the skull. Relax and register your physical impression, the poise of the total skull. Imagine for a moment the structural architecture that you know underlies this feeling. All of the joint relationships throughout the body structure refer directly to the body poise because together they create it. The fluid and membrane of the soft tissue push and pull distinctively.

Now bring your attention to the rhythm of your breath. The breathing rhythm subtly nods the head (rocking of the occipital condyles on the superior articular facets of the atlas).

Wipe your focus clean and pick up the arterial pulsation in the scalp. It should be easy to identify. Listen to it for a while, then wipe your focus clean once again and listen for the craniosacral respiratory impulse. The CRI is palpated as a widening and shortening, then a narrowing and lengthening of the skull. It can be deduced from the pendular motion in your relaxed elbows as they rock subtly back and forth. Now feel the motion in your scapulae as they float in and out in synch with your elbows. In this way, register the craniosacral rhythm in your body. The use of your tactile proprioceptive pathway amplifies your own subjective joint proprioception. Each phase of cranial flexion or extension normally takes about three seconds. When you have registered the rhythm, feel it without judgement for a few minutes. Then begin to note the amplitude and symmetry of the impulse. Practice switching back and forth among the three rhythms at will, wiping your sentient (perceptive) field clean between perceptions.

Now return to poise without losing the rhythm. From your palpatory vantage, imagine the poise of the entire body architecture as it relates to your tactile impression. This exercise strengthens your intuition.

Practice: **Cranial Rhythm on a Subject**

Sit at the head of the table. Your subject is supine. Cradle your subject's head comfortably in your hands, with the ears between the third and fourth fingers (vault hold). Palpate the cranial rhythm for a minute, your blended hands doing what the head is doing. Suspend your elbows and feel the rhythm in them. Notice that you can feel a slight motion in your own arms and in your pectorals. Now "ride" with the rhythm. Get ahead of it by anticipating it just slightly as it flexes and extends, as though the hands welcome and encourage the motion. Now confront the fulcrum; anticipating the maximum motion, resist the last bit of motion not by pushing but by becoming "immoveable as stone." Confront the edge of each phase and let it push up against the "stone" of your hand. Then let it up, and "welcome" it again, riding for several cycles. Now you are ready to practice the palpation of rhythms at the various listening stations of the body. This is the preliminary skill required for working with the craniosacral system.

Fundamental Principles

Placing Your Hands

When first approaching the craniosacral system, place your hands on the body as quietly as possible, "as a bird alights on a twig, and then grabs hold" (Sutherland). Begin with your hands on rather than in the tissue, resting in the interface between the surface of the skin and the atmosphere, between "self" and "not self." Imagine a water spider perched on the surface tension of the water. Be still and receptive. Keep your eyes open. Relax your arms and shoulders, focus on your proprioceptive circuit, and listen. If you begin your therapeutic interaction with your patient in this way, you will have the wisdom of her body to assist your own. After a short time the proprioceptive tract will extend itself across your sensorimotor cortex and connect with the motor function. This is the long loop.

Projecting into the Body: "Dropping In"

The skeleton, and especially the cranium, is an effective handle on the fluid membrane tissue. When your hands are on the cranium or the spine, "drop" your focus in from the skin, muscle, and bone to the membrane tension beneath, and the fluid pressure within it. By expressing the underlying tone, these subjective indicators can help you to interpret what you feel in the musculoskeleton.

Begin with your touch as light as possible. You can move as deeply and dynamically into the tissue as you want and avoid heavy-handedness, and the reflex of squirming grimace that accompanies it, by knowing the poise of the patient's tissues gained from a moment of proprioceptive palpation. In appreciating the resting state, or neurologic tone, of the patient's tissues you gain valuable information about your patient and also let her know that you won't violate her defenses. This allows her to relax her guard by choice and encourages her to trust your hand, maximizing the benefit of your treatment.

When working deep in the tissues, begin outside of the tension poise and "drop in" to the tension level in the tissue. Tension is a neurologic function, and you can communicate neurologically with the tissue tension pattern by matching it exactly and "locking in" just prior to action. Pause here and wait for the tissue to take you in deeper.

You can also "drop in" to the distal tissues from any station of the body. Extend your palpatory inquiry out into the body. The torso is essentially an aggregate of concentric fluid-filled sacs. When you lock in to the frequency of the craniosacral system and its relationship to the exact tension pattern in the body, the body begins to express itself spontaneously. In helping the patient define himself to himself, you have activated a homeostatic response. This is his neural function. Motion induced in this circumstance will tend to be healing for your patient.

Beginning to End

There is in the body potential inherent motion capable of expressing a pattern of tissue holding. This physiologic motion exists subtly as a vortex in the holding pattern of the tissue and the rhythm, and may be induced into motion. These potentials of motion are inherent and autonomic, and can be induced by the interaction of doctor and patient or patient and self. Begin your touch without pressure. Be quiet and curious, just for a moment, and the pressure and tension inherent to the tissue will come up to greet you and draw you in. If your communication with the patient facilitates her communication with herself, and assists her in organizing herself in a more practical, true, and efficient configuration, then you have done the patient some good beyond the ameliorative.

Dropping in to the Rhythm Fulcrum

Inherent to the concept of biphasic craniosacral motion is that of the fulcrum around which the two phases move or at which they meet. The craniosacral fulcrum is the point at which the flexion phase is complete and the extension phase begins. You may find various asymmetries: flexion vs. extension, right vs. left, this bone or that bone, etc. In addition to attempting to increase directly the range of a limited flexion or extension phase, shift the fulcrum of the rhythm itself to a more balanced point, which will then allow a better balance among all aspects of the motion.

The Listening Stations

The listening stations are the various places on the body where it is natural to place the hands and listen to the inherent motion. The use of the word "listen" in this context implies passivity in your activity. "Float" your hands at the surface and feel for fluid wave patterns, pressure, and membrane tension. Suspend your elbows from your wrists and feel the motion in them. Don't judge or doubt your ability. If you think you feel it, assume that you do feel it. Learn to feel confidence without doubt and without arrogance. Traditional listening stations are:

1. the soles of the feet
2. the dorsum of the feet
3. the calves
4. the thighs
5. the ilia
6. the abdomen
7. the thoracic outlet
8. the thoracic inlet
9. the arms and hands
10. the neck
11. the base of the skull
12. the calvarium

The concept of listening stations is not a dogmatic one. It is appropriate to listen anywhere, but use the stations as an opportunity to listen throughout the body so that you can note relative variations from one station to the next.

Palpation of Rhythms

The various rhythms of the body can be palpated at any station. Learn to recognize the nature of each and to feel it anywhere. Then practice selective focus and "wipe the slate clean" as you shift your attention back and forth from one rhythm to the next. The rhythms most readily palpable are the arterial, respiratory, and CRI. The descriptions below are approximations of normal motions and are offered as guidelines. If you feel something different, trust your perception.

1. **Vascular:** The cardiovascular arterial pulse is characterized as a beat (perceived as motility without mobility) and varies from 40 to 100 beats per minute. Although it is conventionally monitored at the radial, carotid, or femoral arteries, it can be palpated anywhere on the body.

T. J. Bennett, D.C., in the notes of his lectures, derives significance from the fact that the blood vessels in embryogenesis pulsate prior to the development of the heart, and he maintains that the arteriole pulse differs somewhat from the cardiac arterial rhythm. *Gray's Anatomy,* 35th British Edition, comments:

> A more intimate control of the blood flow pattern through the microcirculatory units of the various tissues (vide infra) is provided by the muscular walls of the arterioles and precapillary sphincters (resistance vessels).

This seems to indicate that the resistance vessels modify the nature of the arterial pulse and in doing so mediate between the rhythm of the distribution vessels and that of the exchange vessels (capillaries), which transmit one corpuscle at a time and communicate with the tissue extracellular fluid. Bennett advises that the difference is more easily explained as a qualitative rather than a quantitative one:

> ... [T]he character of the pulse is a much better guide than the number of pulses per minute. The pulse (arteriole) is fine, thready and of low tension.

The arteriole rhythm is usually soft and elastic, lacking the hard edge of the arterial thump, an undulating pulsation that rises and falls gently, like a wave, and is assumed to represent the neurologic function related to blood perfusion. Or it can be vigorous and elastic, not like the "lub-dup" of the arterial pulse, which drops out suddenly under your touch, but like a rising progression of bubbles pressing to the surface and sinking hydraulically back down. This aspect of the vascular rhythm is also interesting in that it can by various means be induced to crescendo in amplitude, followed by decrescendo, and then often by tissue release.

2. **Breathing:** The pneumatic respiration creates a wave that originates in the expansion and contraction of the thoracic cage and diaphragm and travels longitudinally through the body. It can normally be palpated in the limbs as a subtle superior and inferior motion, inducing flexion and extension of the occiput on the atlas, and dorsiflexion and plantarflexion of the feet.

3. **Craniosacral rhythm:** The CRI can be palpated on the head and body as a subtle, bilateral corkscrew wave in response to the rhythmic fluctuation of cerebrospinal fluid within the ventricles. The head and torso widen and narrow, and the limbs rotate laterally and medially around the axes of the long bones. Each phase of craniosacral motion usually takes approximately three seconds, although this may vary from two to five seconds. Therefore, one complete cycle of craniosacral motion—one systolic flexion and one diastolic extension—takes about six seconds, and there are approximately ten cycles per minute (six to twelve are considered normal limits).

Palpating Tissue Tension, Fluid Pressure, and Rhythm

Tissue tension, fluid pressure, and rhythm all exert reciprocal influence on one another. In palpation, it is essential to remain relaxed and not try too hard. Let the impression come to you easily and don't indulge in doubt. Feel your own body. The trick is to allow the proprioceptive system to work without too much interference from the thinking mind. This is the long loop: proprioceptive afferent to motor efferent. The treatment is ideally assisted by the "inner physician" or "innate intelligence" of your patient's nervous system.

Practice: Proprioceptive Palpation at the Listening Stations

Place your hands on the head or body. First tune into the arterial rhythm in the body. It can be felt in any tissue. When you have listened to the arterial rhythm satisfactorily, wipe your impression from your mind and, without moving your hand, feel for the vertical wave of breathing. This one is easy and can be verified visually. Now "wipe the slate clean" again. Feel for the cranial rhythmic impulse as sensed in your wrists and between your fingers. Listen quietly for a moment while remaining completely passive. What does it tell you about the adaptation status of the patient? Relax your arms and shoulders. Then let your attention float up and down the dural tube and through the body. It's easy to imagine. Can you feel subluxations through the tube? With passive proprioception, feel tension and pressure gradients and their influence on the cranial rhythm. Trust your impression. Then tug very gently, almost imperceptibly, on the tissues to gain a further impression of where the tissue is hung up. Again focus your attention down the body. Ask yourself: where would I place a push pin or a piece of tape to create this same pattern of resistance? Remember how easy it is to locate a pull on your shirt. The same principle applies here.

Beginning at the feet, move your hands from station to station in order to compare how the body feels from place to place. At each station feel the arterial and breathing rhythms, the craniosacral rhythm, the subtle tissue tension, and then project your attention up and down the dural tube. Train yourself to feel and to trust your perception in a relaxed and humble way. It's not necessary or even advantageous to try to tell the patient what you feel, because your perception is not elicited for the sake of analysis. It's more useful as a starting place from which to initiate change in the neurologic holding pattern. Whenever a patient asks what you are feeling, pull on their shirt.

Restrictions to Normal Motion

The phenomenon of tension and pressure in distal tissues is actively transmitted through the more passive medium of physiologic motion, or normal motility, as an interference pattern. It's like a reed that sticks up out of the water and superimposes its own pattern on that of the pond. Membrane restrictions can also be sensed via gentle tugging.

There is a variety of factors, both active and passive, which can restrict normal mobility and/or motility, including hard and soft fixations, active inflammations, swollen or hypertrophied tissues, etc. One is the neurologic reconfiguration pattern characteristic of adaptations, as is seen in the AK reactive muscle. There may be relation between this type of adaptive reconfiguring phenomenon and that which Upledger calls an "energy cyst."

Each restriction to unified function represents an individual agenda which presents an active, ongoing stress to the whole system economy. Each creates its own wave pattern which can be palpated through the unified wave of the craniosacral impulse. Each interference wave varies from the CRI in rate, amplitude, and vector. Interference waves can be located and amplified by the process of "wiping the slate clean." Wipe your sentient field blank and passively allow the interference pattern, no matter how vague it may be, to dominate your perception.

Practice: **The Fluidity of Tissue**

The subject is prone. Place three fingers of your palpating hand over the lumbosacral junction. The pressure of your touch should be just light enough for tissue pull. Slowly feel the elasticity of the tissues by tractioning the skin cephalad and then caudal. The cephalad traction will be a push and the caudal traction a pull. Each traction should take about ten seconds. In the first five seconds you should reach the easy limit of tissue stretch. For the second five seconds, continue to exert drag on the tissue. Without increasing your force, you will feel the engagement of the underlying tissue, skin via reciprocal attachment to myofascia to bone to spinal cord. Next hold the traction for a full minute, consistently maintaining your vector of traction without force. Feel the fluid nature of tissue, and the way your wave of push or pull can be subtly pushed or pulled through the tensile and hydraulic medium of the body tissues all the way to the fluid environment of the subdural spine. You can feel the whole spinal structure, hard to soft to fluid, "crawl" like a snake.

Now push a wave up toward the head and follow the wave as it travels all the way up the spine. Hold your traction until you feel its effects reach all the way up to the head. Next, as you pull the sacrum into flexion, feel the tension change in the spinal cord as you traction the intervertebral discs and the coccyx moves anterior. In this configuration, the spinal column lengthens while the spinal cord is allowed to relax. Hold the pull and feel the wave travel through the fluid medium.

This exercise will familiarize you with the way neural tissue exhibits the behavioral properties of a highly viscous fluid, and it will train your touch to effectively reach down into the matter of the spinal tract itself. As the wave travels up the spine, can you feel the location of subluxations and fixations?

Interpreting the Craniosacral Rhythm

The Cranial Respiratory Impulse is palpated at the head and listening stations of the body and evaluated in terms of frequency, amplitude, symmetry, and character at the various locales. Frequency and amplitude of the cranial rhythm allow us to comprehend our patient's summary status in the general equation of stress adaptation. If the amplitude is slightly increased and the rhythm is reasonably normal and symmetrical, this may indicate a high stress demand which presently does not present a serious and immediate threat to the patient's overall vitality. The adaptation thusfar is probably reasonably successful and the adaptive reserves are probably adequate to meet the demand. It is as though the system is "pushing through" a challenge.

The febrile state often increases the frequency of the CRI. A doubling of frequency with a faint amplitude may represent a meningeal restriction due to active or past inflammation, with the adaptive vitality of the subject thusfar, but not necessarily forever, holding its own. A decrease of both factors may indicate a less successful response to the demands of life, indicating a more serious need for treatment and possibly a longer prognosis. In coma patients, both frequency and amplitude of the CRI are substantially depressed. A lack of symmetry in the presence of normal frequency and amplitude indicates somatic restriction, such as fixation, active inflammation, etc., possibly within the cranium, but also possibly in distal body tissues.

A phenomenon can be observed in denervated tissue, such as exists in the body of a victim of spinal cord severance. Denervated tissue, which lacks the modulating restraint of the CRI, pulsates at a frequency of 25-30 cycles per minute. In one quadriplegic patient who had suffered partial severance at C5 subsequent to receiving a bullet in the neck, the craniosacral rhythm was palpable throughout most of his body, with the exception of his left leg below the knee. The significance of this remains a question, but this patient has since willfully contracted his left quadriceps muscle.

Variation of craniosacral motion from place to place in the body contributes to our diagnostic impression of the patient and at the same time is taken without regard to diagnosis to represent restriction or fixation of the tissue; in other words, to determine not "what" but "where" and to what degree.

Releasing Restrictions: Basic Concepts of Tissue Release

Hard and soft tissue holding patterns of both long and short duration can be released by the body. In some situations, releasing restrictions works best when it comes as an autonomic decision on the part of the patient's system, rather than by the doctor working against the patient's autonomic will. This may seem contradictory to the concept of being a doctor and "fixing" the patient, but it actually leaves us lots of room in which to interact with the patient to her greatest benefit, by providing a situation in which the autonomic self can successfully complete its "unfinished business." The autonomic body cannot be made to change against its will. It is usually in its predicament because, given the options, it has chosen its best bet. Steal its adaptation without restoring proper function and you may force it into an adaptation pattern of increased complexity and consequence.

Membrane releases by shifting into a more advantageous configuration. The autonomically deliberate shift of tissue is something that the patient understands innately. In the shifting of tissues there is fluid movement as well and this can be homeostatic to pressure gradients in the body.

Borborygmus

Borborygmus, the rumbling of gas in the intestines, frequently accompanies tissue release. In this context, it doesn't seem to have much to do with digestive function. The reciprocal tension relationship of the mesentery to the rest of the body structure probably accounts for this evidence of shifting. Patients will frequently make an embarrassed remark about either being hungry or having just eaten. The synchronicity of touch with borborygmy sounds is not incidental.

Direct and Indirect Release

Direct release implies a corrective effort which directly counters the distortion. A right posterior subluxation is adjusted anteriorly to the left. A tight muscle is stretched. Indirect release implies a corrective effort that commences by exaggerating the distortion.

We are all familiar with direct techniques. Indirect techniques often work by allowing the organism to express itself, tolerantly encouraging the distortion, following it, and then seeing what the organism chooses to do next. Let it do whatever it wants, with one exception: don't let it backtrack. This is the foundation strategy of the indirect technique that proves so useful in meningeal adjustment.

Sometimes in approaching the shape of release a patient will feel extreme discomfort, even though the distortion doesn't seem that dramatic. In this situation, push the line but not the limit. Stop for a moment on the edge of the discomfort and tell him that you won't go past that point. I tell my patients that with their permission and within their tolerance, I will continue. Permission given, I remind them once more that I'll stop at any time they want me to, and then I continue in. Most people will relax completely at this point, which really helps range of motion.

Energetic Release

Because "energy" is a much-abused and often esoteric term, it is a subject of potential controversy and ridicule. It can't be seen and is difficult to objectify. Anyone can claim to have "moved some energy" without having to verify the results and often without apparent benefit. Despite these problems, when all is said and done, energy is behavior, and behavior is really the point. The task is similar to that of proving color to the colorblind.

We can learn to perceive and even demonstrate what we cannot by nature prove.

The hands, by design, communicate superbly. The nervous system is specifically designed for communication and ubiquitously pervades the tissues. It communicates best; that's what it is and what it does. It is specifically responsive to behavior and also to thought. If you are cynical, or if you simply possess a healthy skepticism, suspend your doubt for a day or two and experiment with this. You are, of course, free to resume your doubt at the conclusion of the experiment. Neurologic tissue responds willingly to thought, but like any willful entity, it doesn't respond as readily to linear, "left-brain" commands as it does to more pictorial and generative "right-brain" visualization. It responds best of all to attentive listening, a thought process of some subtlety, skill, and power. To listen to the autonomic nervous system of your patient with your proprioceptive ability is to appreciate, perhaps as fully as is possible, the meaning of "innate intelligence."

Many of us routinely use "mind over matter" as a practice-building strategy and use visualization to manifest our aspirations to a high degree of specificity. Thought (intent) is the basis of action. The "placebo effect" is another tip-of-the-iceberg example of this most powerful imaging potential. The willful therapeutic application of this principle is worth exploring for both the doctor and the patient. So frequently in our desire to satisfy requirements of objectivity and reproducibility we reduce our own potential to the lowest common denominator, denying ourselves the unity of balance (homeostasis).

Often this type of work can attract people with tendencies toward naivety, contributing to the somewhat understandable public perception of the subtle as "flaky." On the other hand, there exists in our society a wholesale dismissal of all that is subtle in unbalanced favor of the "objective." Because life is to each of us predominantly a subjective experience, and because so much of this experience is "subconscious" and autonomic, the discounting of the subtle represents a profound oversight.

It's interesting that one aspect of the human mind demands rigorous objectivity while another aspect may have little regard for the concept and prefers to be approached with a respect for the subjective. By cementing our approach in a foundation of orthopedics, objective findings, and a thorough understanding of physiology, we are allowed freedom to interact with our patient without losing our footing. Neither dichotomy nor contradiction, but both sides of a coin.

Energetic release of tissue patterns can be active or passive, involving gross movement or subtle movement, or no apparent movement.

Proprioceptive Listening

The human nervous system behaves in ways similar to our conscious experience. If you've ever had a friend who offered unsolicited advice or chronic devil's advocacy, full of rationales and options in response to any difficulty you might be having, you may have felt overwhelmed by the friendship and probably learned to avoid revealing any problem to this person. You may have rebelled against the unwanted advice even to your own disadvantage. Another friend might be skilled at lending an understanding ear, offering only occasional observations, a question, or a supportive comment, and it will likely be this encouraging friend that you seek out in a time of need. In the presence of this friend, comfortable that you can be yourself, you spill all your beans. Maybe afterwards some things don't seem so bad after all, and maybe some things even seem funny. This friend, in allowing you a quiet and sympathetic forum, helped you to reach your own conclusions and to successfully adapt to the demands of the time.

In this spirit, listening to the neurologic rhythms and refraining from stimulating the patient with your perceptions and remedial advice (treatment) can be a powerful therapeutic mode. The recognition of intelligence in neurologic tissue is not pathetic fallacy (in which human traits are attributed to inanimate objects). It is apparent that the nervous system is no dummy and knows when it is being listened to, and appreciates that quiet and accepting forum. I have had the experience at times of working with a patient intently, trying with all my effort to effect a real change by various means, adjusting, myofascial work, etc., and suddenly becoming aware of the tension in my own body and in the situation, then relaxing, softening my grip, and sitting down to listen to the neural rhythm. The body comes alive, pulsating, processing, revealing a mind of its own. Suddenly, sometimes within a few seconds, sometimes after a few minutes, the tissues shift, soften, let go. Fixations release. The indicators clear. My advice might even have been the right advice, but the system wanted to make its own choice. That this autonomic response is deliberate will be obvious to anyone who experiences it. This is the power of communication, for which all nervous systems and all people hunger.

Direction of Energy

The direction of energy or "V-spread" as taught by Upledger is a fundamental cornerstone of craniosacral technique. The V-spread can best be described as a direct application of mind to matter, or more specifically, to brain. Physics tells us that matter and energy are substantially the same; matter is slowed-down energy and energy is speeded-up matter. The V-spread allows us to apply this principle to the therapeutic benefit of our patient.

Practice: V-Spread

Place your hands on either side of a restricted tissue and imagine a current of flow that runs between them. The term V-spread comes from the image of the current traveling between the V's formed by the junction at the base of two fingers of either hand. The current can be DC or AC. After a few moments you will feel a pulsation (the neurovascular or arteriole rhythm) that crescendos and then decrescendos, followed by a palpable shifting or softening of the tissues.

The V-spread can be applied to hard or soft tissue, through the plane of an intracranial membrane, to a sutural restriction, or a fixated vertebra or peripheral joint. It can also be applied to an area of acute pain, often with noticeable results.

Perhaps the use of imagination to influence material reality, like the fact of existence itself, cannot be rationally justified. We will have to be satisfied with its clinical utility. It might make us rethink the meaning of the Biblical myth that God created man in His own "image."

Energetic interaction is by its nature communicative. Its therapeutic power is inherent to the organism of the patient and helps him to better organize his function.

Still Point

Another cornerstone of craniosacral technique is the still point. The still point feels like a "shutting down" of the craniosacral rhythm and can be interpreted as representing a neurologic opportunity for processing autonomic change. The still point can occur intrinsically or can be induced extrinsically. To induce a still point in your patient, gently resist one phase of craniosacral motion while allowing the other phase. In a few moments to a few minutes you'll feel the system begin to rhythmically disorganize and "wobble," followed by the still point, which may itself last moments or minutes. The patient will experience the still point as being quietly and subtly pleasurable. Children are especially suitable for still point induction, and it can often be used to gain their trust.

The still point is appropriate at any phase of treatment, but may be induced either near the beginning of treatment, where it serves to encourage receptivity in the patient's nervous system, or at the conclusion of treatment, where it serves to allow the integration of changes elicited in the neurostructure during the visit. It also tends to smooth any rough edges that the patient may feel upon emerging from treatment, thus preparing him for reentry into the functional state.

It seems unlikely that the still point could represent a de facto cessation of CSF production. Rather than suspending the perfusion of CSF, maybe the system simply turns off the pump pulsation, allowing the creation of CSF by streaming ionic diffusion across the choroid plexus in equilibrium with the bulk flow of the arachnoid drain. During the still point, think of the CSF as gently streaming.

Figure 24: Hand position for still point induction

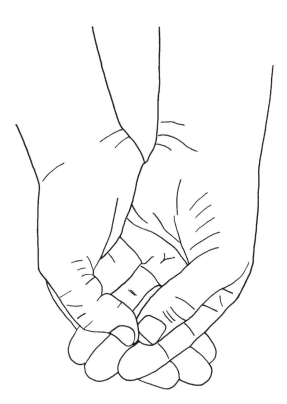

Practice: Still Point Induction on the Cranium: CV4

Cradle the head with cupped hands so that the temporal mastoid processes rest in your thenar eminences and your fingers extend caudally along the neck. Touch your thumbs together and listen for the cranial rhythm at the mastoids. On cranial flexion the mastoids approximate, on extension they separate. You can feel this motion at your elbows and in your triceps. Follow the motion of flexion by subtly compressing your thenars together to accompany the mastoids as they approximate. Now gently but firmly resist the separation of the mastoids as cranial extension begins. Don't push the mastoids together, simply become as immoveable as stone and don't allow the mastoids to move apart. Again follow the flexion as the next cycle begins, and once again become immoveable in response to extension. After a few cycles you will feel a quickened pulsation as the craniosacral system begins to disorganize, and then the rhythm will stop. After a time it will begin anew. You may want to resist the mastoids in moving apart for a few cycles to allow it to build up some momentum. Then allow the extension to express itself and continue to monitor the CRI for a few more cycles. Evaluate the motion for rate, amplitude, and symmetry. The still point may be repeated several times if you wish.

Still Point Induction at the Feet

Sit at the feet, relax your shoulders, and cup both heels gently, allowing them to rest in your palms. Mold your hands to the shape of the heels without grasping. Feel in your arms for the craniosacral motion as it rotates the feet. On flexion the feet rotate apart (eversion) and on extension they move together (inversion). Allow a couple of cycles, then follow extension (inversion) to its end and resist its return by becoming immoveable. Again, you will feel the throbbing wobble of disorganization followed by a stop. Treat the still point as you did at the head, allowing it to build up pressure before permitting flexion to resume.

The still point can be induced anywhere in the body, at any time, by passively resisting the craniosacral motion.

Unwinding

Spontaneous Release by Positioning

Spontaneous release by positioning is another concept that comes to us from osteopathy. It serves as a foundation for applications that are profound and have yet to be fully explained. When a person is injured, he spontaneously tenses. If the trauma has sufficient impact, which may be physical, mental, emotional, etc., it can become locked into the holding pattern of the tissue (potential energy). This whole-body response is registered into the neurostructure partially as the configuration of body position at the time of impact and partially as the "seizure" response of the body to the impact and the vector of impact as it travels into the tissue. If the configuration can be recaptured (or reconjured), the body can be given the chance to release this configuration of holding and free up some autonomic reserve. Upledger refers to the traumatically induced holding pattern as an "energy cyst."

There are several applications of spontaneous release by positioning in therapeutics, including "strain-counterstrain," osteopathic "muscle energy" techniques, and craniosacral unwinding.

Unwinding

Unwinding is inherent corrective physiologic motion that can be induced from the nervous system. It is spontaneous release by positioning in which the position keeps changing. The unwinding process often seems like nothing and can at other times be dramatic. Learn to "listen" for the tendency of the body to bend or rotate, and follow the tendency. Also, learn to project your palpation into the body as the motion occurs so that the movement relates the head and neck to the rest of the body. This is the beginning of the unwinding process. You may also notice some tendency toward cranial unwinding when tractioning the cranial membranes.

Unwinding can begin in any limb or from any body part. As you feel the almost incidental motion begin, feel the rest of the body from your station, relating the limb in its motion to the dural tube, the other limbs, the head and neck, and torso.

Practice: Unwinding

Sit at the head. The subject lies supine with her shoulders to the head of the table. Holding her head in one hand, place the other hand over the frontal bone and lightly grab hold of it. Palpate rhythm and tension for a moment. Now let the head move slowly, arbitrarily. The arbitrary motion, if palpated, proves capable of expressing the will of the neck. A body in motion propels the first three dimensions through the fourth (time) and each other. Project your feeling down the dural tube and into the whole body as the head moves. Follow the motion wherever it seems to want to go, but gently and firmly resist any tendency of the motion to backtrack. This presents the organism with the opportunity to select a new behavior, helping to free it from the dilemma of pattern fixation.

Now stand at the foot of the table, with the subject lying supine, head on the table. Gently hold her heels in your cupped hands, lift her legs easily, and slowly begin to move her legs back and forth a bit. Feel the tension of the legs and their expression of dural torsion. Project your attention to the lumbar cistern and the spray of the cauda equina. Listen for the will of the organism. You may feel like lifting the legs, or they may both swing to one side or separate, and then one may lift. Listen for natural stopping points, when the organism needs to pause and process. These pauses are characterized by still points, in which the craniosacral rhythm pauses. Another way to recognize these stopping points is by the sensation of "plugging in," in which you may feel a movement of energy, which might feel like a warmth accompanied by a mild electromagnetic tingle, or a feeling similar to that of being in a magnetic field. Some practitioners report sensations in their own body, such as in the limbs or feet. One person reports that he always feels tingling in his ears, face, and temples at still points. Focusing on this feeling of being "plugged in" can help you stay on the right track through the unwinding progress. After a while it will become second nature. Once again, if you feel the tendency to

Figure 25: *Unwinding*

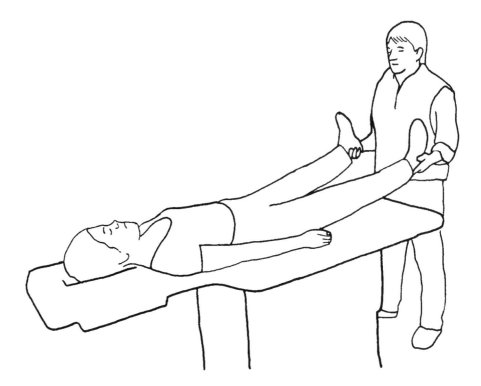

backtrack in the patient, become an immovable obstacle to this, allowing the organism to choose a new way out.

Try unwinding from one arm, using the long-loop function to relate the limb to the dural tube, the cranium and sacrum, and other limbs. Trust the impulse to lift the head, or to move to another station. As you practice unwinding more and more, you will feel increasingly confident in the rightness of a certain movement, position, resting place, when to allow and when to resist.

I learned something special from many hours of unwinding the quadriplegic man mentioned previously. His body would not allow the passage of the ascending afferent response to moving a limb; the signal seemed to bounce back and ricochet into the other limbs. Thus to lift his left arm would cause his legs to fire off and kick to the right, strongly enough to flop his body toward the edge of the mattress he was lying on. I found that if I moved his body slowly enough, painstakingly slow, his nervous system would accept continual motion without setting off, and each limb when moved that slowly for an hour at a time would seem to take on a life of its own, stopping at certain points and changing direction.

The techniques and styles of unwinding all derive from the clinical process of trained listening and activation of the "long loop," which helps the doctor to facilitate the patient's own best need. Spinal unwinding is perfectly chiropractic. It works well blended with general technique, when the patient doesn't know you're using it. Let the neck unwind for one minute and it's butter in your hands. And the hands, having learned to better recognize the neck in its relationship to the brain and body, give a more profound adjustment. Through reciprocal tension and biomechanics you can lever your adjustment in with other body structures or spinal levels.

Practice: Unwinding the Thorax

You can unwind the thoracic spine and cage with the patient supine or prone. Blend your hand on the sternum or back, feel the rhythm, meet the tension, and drop in. As you move in, follow the natural torsion of the tissues to their conclusion. There is the limit of that tissue pattern; along with the limitation of the other phase or range of motion, it defines the pattern. Follow the tissue distortion and allow it to do anything it wants, but if it begins to backtrack, become immovable and don't let it. This will require it to choose a new behavior and may induce a permanent change in the tissue tension.

By tolerant recognition of the pattern and identification of its parameters to the signalling system, the autonomic corrective process can begin to be activated. A small bit of perceptible good can prove to be of significant benefit to a patient because you have moved the fulcrum of his pendulum toward a new balance. Unwinding can initiate a process that continues well beyond the time of the patient's visit to your office.

Cup the head in one hand and lay your other hand on the sternum. Encourage your subject to give his head to you as dead weight. Now extend your perception down the tube for a second and let your hand move the head slowly and arbitrarily. Become an immovable barrier to any tendency for the motion to backtrack.

Compress your hands together and feel the way the discs accommodate. Push that limit slightly and see if there's any unwinding potential in there. Now traction your hands apart, the slower the better. You're testing the way the tissue crawls as the discs and meninges open. As the neck lengthens, does it want to flex or extend, to the right or left?

Is the whole thing really that easy, can we really get right in there? The answer is a qualified yes. The trick, of course, is developing and keeping your focus. And the patient must let you in.

The Dural Tube

The Vertebral Canal

Although anatomists report some variation, the dura as it descends from the foramen magnum does not, in most people, attach to the ring of the atlas, but adheres again at C2/C3 and from there drops to the

Figure 26: *Denticulate ligament*

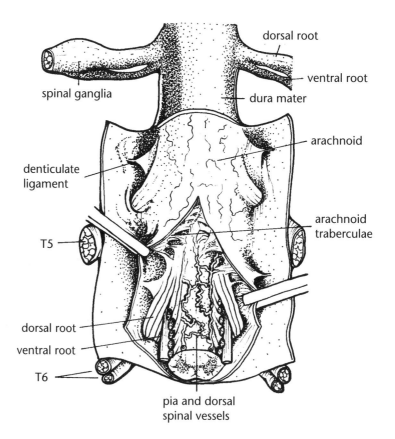

dorsal root

ventral root

dura mater

spinal ganglia

arachnoid

denticulate ligament

arachnoid traberculae

T5

dorsal root

ventral root

T6

pia and dorsal spinal vessels

sacrum without substantial adhesion to the vertebral canal except via the dural attachments at the sleeves of the nerve roots. For this reason it is considered semi-freely gliding. As it glides, it exerts traction on the dural sleeves.

The spinal cord itself attaches to the inside of the dura throughout its cascade alternately by the ventral and dorsal roots and the denticulate ligaments, strands of epipial tissue that reach laterally through the CSF medium and anchor the pia mater, and thus the spinal tissue, to the inside of the dura.

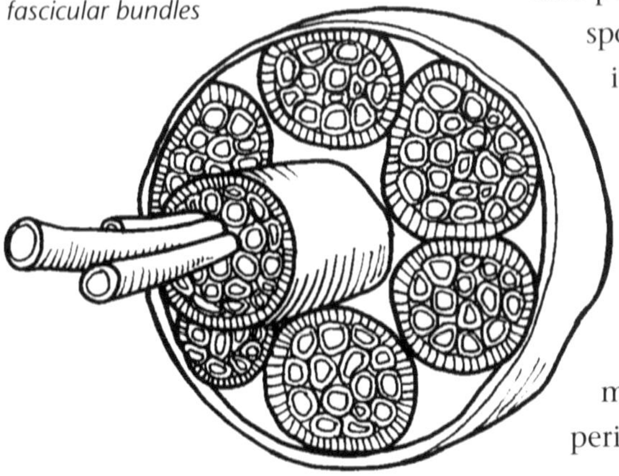

Figure 27: Peripheral fascicular bundles

The spinal cord white matter is segmentally arranged into anterior, lateral, and posterior columns, divided by the sulci, which correspond to fascial compartments in the body. Each column is then subdivided in a homuncular layout of fibers—cervical, thoracic, lumbar, and in the posterior columns, sacral—each containing the nerve fascicles, themselves ensheathed in epineurium and perineurium. The fascicles create the spinal nerve roots. Electrical cable is bundled in much the same way. The neurofascicular bundles transmit the craniosacral motion through the spinal cord and out through the peripheral nerves to all somatic structures.

The epineurium of each peripheral nerve is linearly contiguous with the capsule of its target muscle and literally enmeshes it. This vector contributes strongly to the transmission of CNS motility to the musculoskeletal body. Within the neurofascial mesh are proprioceptive bodies. They are receptive not only to somatic position and resting set points but also to rhythm. At the proper set point for each muscle at rest or in motion, the rhythm is inherently harmonious with the brain rhythm.

Magoun relates his finding of a groove in the vertebral canal, posteriorly in the lordotic cervical and lumbar areas and anteriorly in the thoracic spine, indicating that the dura is in frequent contact with the canal as it stretches over the spinal curves. This underscores that the expression of CNS physiologic rhythm is a dynamic between the fluid impulse and the tensile forces of membrane.

Atlas and Upper Cervical Mechanism

The exemption of the atlas ring from the dura frees it somewhat but not completely from the structural concerns of the body in favor of some of the "higher" skeletal and neuromuscular functions, which are concerned with vision and turning the head to look, smell, speech, hearing, facial expression, equilibrium, and eating; in other words, to provide the upper cervical neuro-musculoskeletal accompaniment to the cranial nerve special senses and to self-expression. This, of course, is a neonatal behavior.

The upper cervical mechanism can be considered in the prone and supine positions. Prone, the atlas is flexed on C2, and hovers in suspension above the axis odontoid on the sling of the transverse ligament. Supine, the atlas is extended on C2, and pendulates beneath an odontoid fulcrum.

Palpation and Mobilization of the Sacrum

The sacrum can be palpated with the subject either supine or prone. According to DeJarnette, when the subject is supine the weight-bearing function of the sacroiliac articulation tends to remain engaged, thereby allowing a natural approach to the ilium as it relates to and influences the sacrum. With the subject prone the sacrum can somewhat disengage from that relationship and can float. Now it's more fundamentally in relationship with the occiput (i.e., craniosacral/neurologic function) through the tube. Of course both functions of the sacrum exist in all postures.

Palpating the Dural Tube

The dural tube can be palpated from any locale on the body. At first, learn to palpate it from directly in line with it: from the head and from the sacrum and the feet. From the occiput or parietals or shoulders you can, with an easy pull, engage the inherent tension in the dural membrane. You can feel subluxations and fixations down the tube. Upledger calls this "taking a walk down the tube." After you are comfortable from these vantages, practice checking into the dura while palpating at any listening station and from any limb. You can feel it, innately.

Vertebral Restrictions

The vertebral segments by virtue of their segmentation graphically represent the body to the brain. The autonomic system reads the body configuration as a natural expression of itself. Fixation in the broadest terms represents a loss of dynamic, in which the potential to adapt is partially usurped by the holding patterns of current and past adaptation. It as though the chronic adaptations, while useful in their way, are taking up RAM memory, or functional reserve. This leaves less neurologic availability for facing the current challenges.

Because each intervertebral foramen is bivertebral, the dural sleeves are by design susceptible to torsional forces that relate directly and reciprocally to structural dynamics. The sleeve, which attaches to the hemiforamina of the adjacent vertebrae, is subject to distortion in planes perpendicular to the longitudinal orientation of the dural sheath. Remember that the torsible dural ports provide the sole anchor for the descending dura. Their distortion interacts with the longitudinal orientation of the dura (and body) to create pinching vortices of tension in the craniosacral system which reach right in and impose themselves on the fascicles of the spinal cord.

The Electrical Consequence of Spinal Torsion

The phenomenon of nerve root torsion and compression lies at the heart of the chiropractic model. D.D. Palmer first proposed that neural transmission was significantly impeded by subluxation forces. This seems especially feasible when we consider that the entire fluid milieu of the nervous system expresses the electrical charge of neurologic activity. Electrical transmission itself can be explained in terms of fluid dynamics (voltage = pressure) and is influenced by the vector alignment (flow) of electrons in the fluid conductor, the diameter and length of the conductor, temperature, etc. Dural torsion at the intervertebral foramen creates a pressure backup and interferes with the streaming of electrons through the fluid medium and tissue. It also tends to increase resistance in the form of heat.

Palmer described nerve "energy" as electrical, but the cultural concept of electricity at that time was crude. It is apparent that while neural activity shows characteristics of being a "surge" phenomenon, like the raw, unrefined power that is delivered to appliances, it also demonstrates specifically defined behavioral characteristics closely resembling electronic function, somewhat like a modem. In other words, the nerve is trophic but even more significantly it is communicative.

The electronic is distinguished from the electrical in the sophistication of its organization and the subtlety of its charge. It is the organization of neurologic behavior that communicates specificity to the body systems, thereby maximizing successful adaptation.

It is similar to the transmission of data over a modem. The mode of connecting is simple and binary, requires energy, and closely resembles all other connecting behavior, but once the connection is established the transmission is complex, specific, and both digital and analogue. And it undergoes transformation from form to form (word processor to ASCII to electronic signal to

ASCII and possibly to another word-processing format; willful impulse to electrical impulse to neurochemical transmission to behavior) without alteration of its essence, which is its organization. It is the content of the message that justifies the sophistication of this organizational effort.

The Facilitated Segment

D.D. Palmer suggested that chronic subluxation patterns (and disease) are due to trauma, poison (including autotoxicity), or autosuggestion. The concept of the **facilitated segment** has a similar basis. It implies that a somatic or visceral component is actively interacting with the nervous system in a way that presents chronic stress demands and continually impedes optimal function. Although subluxation patterns are not the cause of disease, the state of the body does manifest itself in structural terms at all times. The whole is always greater than the sum of its parts.

There are physical holding or breakdown patterns that consistently transmit interference signals into the afferent nervous system. These patterns transmit themselves to the brain segmentally and hierarchically. The facilitated segment is a facilitation of the afferent pathway that inputs to the brain, stimulating response. If for any reason satisfactory communication is denied to the origin of the signal, the signal is kept in holding storage, like a computer billboard service might store a transmission until you finally turn on your modem.

The model of the facilitated segment includes the vertebral component as well as the peripheral and core components as they exist, simultaneously. It may reside primarily in any body structure or relationship of body structures. It may present a significant or minor challenge. It may seem insignificant for ten years and then become major. It may remain a minor concern for the life of the organism. It may lie quiescent at times and flare up only in times of specific stress demands. Anything is possible.

The facilitated segment can be palpated through the meningeal tube. It is the subluxation-fixation complex and includes the components "above" and "below" the IVF as well.

Mobilizing the Tube

The dural tube can be mobilized by traction, vertebral adjustment, "V-spread," and unwinding. The influence on the meningeal tube by the adjustment of vertebra is via the dural attachments at the ports of the intervertebral foramen. If an adjustment fails to hold, it is worth considering the membrane tension as a possible influence. Use gentle traction from the occipital base or the parietal station to mobilize minor restrictions. You can recheck by palpation.

Practice: Traction of the Sacrum and Dural Tube

Sit comfortably at the pelvis. Slip your hand under the sacrum from below and cradle it, fingers pointed cephalic. Slip your other hand under the fifth lumbar from the side, fingers parallel to the sacral base. Sit for a moment and register the rhythm and tension at this area. Now slowly begin to pull your sacral hand caudal to traction the sacrum away from the fifth lumbar. When the sacrum and L5 have softened, continue your pull, now projecting up the dural tube towards the upper cervical attachment. Practice naming the levels where you can feel dural tube restrictions. Calm and steady traction here will begin to free the tube. You may be inclined to allow some slow unwinding motion to occur.

The Diaphragms:
Cross Restrictions to the Longitudinal Orientation of the Musculoskeletal System

The longitudinal orientation to the musculoskeletal system between the top of the head and the feet is contradicted at the feet, pelvic diaphragm, respiratory diaphragm, thoracic inlet, cranial base, and scalp. Each of these cross restrictions is a natural location for a torsional vortex in the body. Any torsion palpated at these landmarks can be treated to improve symmetry in the reciprocal tension system. Neutralizing the body diaphragms minimizes their influence in distorting the cranial membrane and maximizes the efficacy of your cranial adjustment.

Craniosacral Flexion

The flexion phase of the cranial rhythm, which causes the skull to widen and shorten, might also be seen as a functional cross restriction to longitudinal orientation, especially when fixated. Extension, which lengthens and narrows the skull, tractions the cranial membranes longitudinally.

Practice: Diaphragm Release

Sit at the pelvis. Place one hand under the lumbosacral junction and the other hand over the pubic bone. Listen for a minute or so and drop your focus in, then begin to approximate your hands, pushing them slowly together to slightly compress the pelvic ring. As you continue to compress, your hands will begin to rotate slightly in relation to one another. Follow the rotation without allowing the tissue to backtrack. When you feel release, repeat the compression

Figure 28: *Pelvic
diaphragm release*

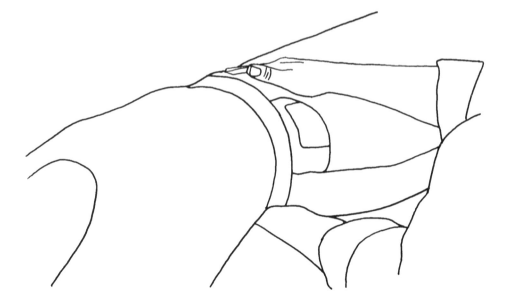

and check for balance and symmetry. This procedure can be repeated several
times if necessary.

Now sit at the thoracic outlet and place one hand under the thoracic spine
and the other over the chest, half over the stomach and half over the xiphoid
and sternum. Compress your hands over the respiratory diaphragm and follow
the torsion, passively resisting any backtracking but allowing the tissue to
choose any other option. Recheck for symmetry and balance. When you are
satisfied, move to the thoracic inlet.

Figure 29: *Thoracic
diaphragm release*

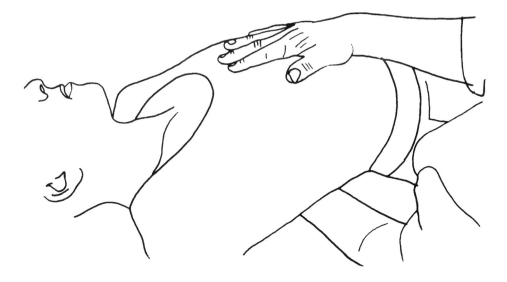

With one hand beneath the cervical-dorsal junction and the other over the sternal notch, approximate your hands and follow the torsion as you have done at the lower two diaphragms. Again, encourage the tissue to choose a new pattern of behavior. You are relying on the homeostatic mechanism innate to each body.

Figure 30: Thoracic inlet release

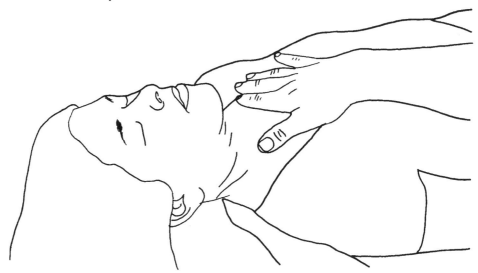

Occipital Decompression

Having cleared the three torso diaphragms, you are now ready to proceed to the occipital cranial base. Cup the head in your hands and place your fingers

Figure 31: Occipital decompression

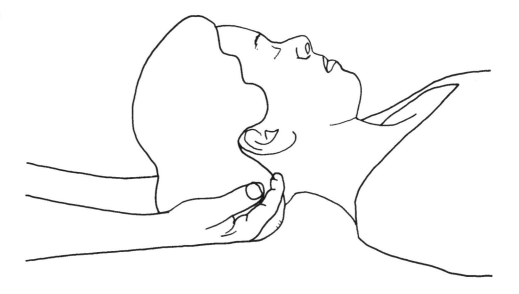

under the occiput pointing straight into the ring of the atlas. Allow the head to relax onto your fingers until the suboccipital musculature lets you in against the posterior ring. Wait here until you feel release. Then use your two pinkies to reach up to either side of the external occipital crest and gently traction the occiput away from the spine. A more forceful traction is in relationship to the lower cervicals and the torso and will tend to drag the upper cervical mechanism together as a unit. A delicate traction separates the occiput from the atlas and axis. Continue to traction down the dural tube.

Figure 32: *Hand position for occipital decompression*

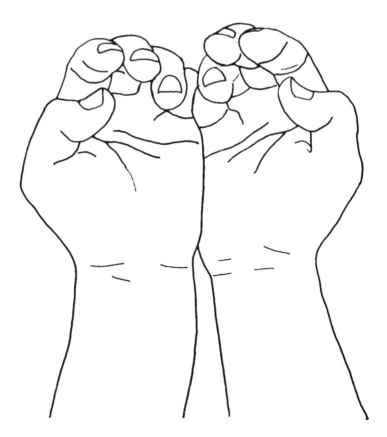

Cranial Adjusting

*I*n adjusting the cranium, it is important that sutural fixations be released, and beyond that the bones are used primarily as handles on the membrane tension and the fluid pressure that it contains. Develop a palpatory sensitivity to cranial mobility and motility as your main indicator, and use the inherent homeostatic tendency of the organism to assist you in the correction. Some restrictions will release spontaneously and others will not because the organism is using them, for better or worse, for its own adaptive purposes. In the course of restoring homeostasis to the body, you may encounter configurations that express holding and breakdown patterns of all types, including adaptations to lifestyle behavior, emotional fixations, past injuries, etc., and it may be necessary to deal with these real-life issues in order to gain adaptive reserve. The patient might benefit from a referral to a competent professional in such a case.

The guidelines provided here are not intended to serve as the primary source of training in craniosacral technique. It is recommended that you seek direct instruction from a trained professional. These pages will therefore serve best as a review. Remember to use only gentle force when applying the principles of cranial bone and membrane technique.

With your hands on the cranium, "drop in" to the underlying membrane tension and CSF pressure. Develop trust in your palpation skills as your main indicator. Then apply traction to the cranial bone to open the sutures. When you feel the sutures separate, continue your traction and allow the membranes to shift. Underlying each hard tissue release is a soft tissue release. Continually extend your inquiry deep and out into the body and you will be rewarded with information about your patient that does not readily lend itself to verbal articulation and is not available by any other means. The interrelatedness of all things can be palpated as you go.

If the sutures are fixated and don't easily release, apply "direction of energy" technique (V-spread) until they do. This usually works.

The Upledger protocol of cranial adjustment is organized according to the underlying membrane attachments. Sit comfortably at the head. It helps to keep in mind Sutherland's advice that your touch should begin "as a bird alights on a twig, and then grabs hold." As you develop your "long loop" function, palpation and adjustment will begin to blend into one.

Begin with still point induction on the temporal mastoids. Now you are ready to begin to traction the cranial membranes.

Figure 33: Relation of surface to bones

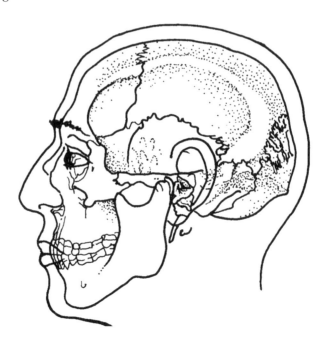

Vertical Intracranial Membrane Release: Falx

Practice: Frontal Lift
(Anterior-Posterior Cranial Membrane Traction)

In the neonatal skull there are two frontal bones separated by a central **metopic suture**, which in all but a few cases fuses in childhood and is obliterated in the adult. Because cranial bone motion is a reflection of the bilateral, rhythmic CSF "urging" beneath, the frontal bone can be palpated as though the metopic suture persists.

Place your hands so that your fingers span the frontal bone just above the orbits. Your fifth fingers should be just inside the articulation with the parietal and the greater wing of the sphenoid (pterion). As you alight onto the bone, mentally "magnetize" your fingers to maximize their grip on the bone. Now begin to apply traction directly anterior (toward the ceiling) and wait for the sutures to disengage. Your "suggestion" of lift is as potent as the physical force you apply, and the development of this skill of mental suggestion will be useful to you again and again in working with the craniosacral system. Continue your traction, feeling the tensity of the falx cerebri, and allow the membranes to shift. The weight of the head accomplishes the adjustment. When you feel the tissue soften, move the bone slightly and explore its range of motion. Then let the bone float back into place and recheck by palpation.

Figure 34: *Frontal lift*

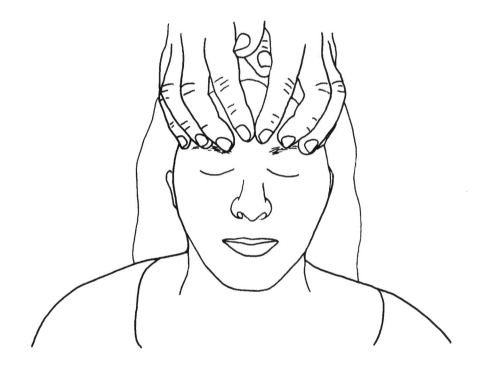

Practice: **Parietal Lift**
(Superior-Inferior Cranial Membrane Traction)

The parietals relate directly to the sagittal sinus beneath the sagittal suture. It is here that the arachnoid granulations drain CSF into the venous blood via bulk flow. The parietals can also be utilized to traction the straight sinus via the falx cerebri.

Begin with your fingers spread along the temporoparietal suture just superior to the temporal bones. Because the beveled temporal bones overlap the parietals, exert some medial pressure on the parietals to disengage them from underneath the temporals and then traction straight superior until you feel the sutures release. Continue to traction the falx from the foramen magnum, and allow the membranes to shift. Sometimes the release comes on one side first, and then the other side balances out. You can gently pump the straight sinus by easing your traction and then resuming it again a few times. When you feel the tissue soften, move the bones back and forth a little to test their mobility. At this point, you can also cross your thumbs across the sagittal suture and stretch it a bit, gently pumping it a few times. When you are satisfied that release has been obtained, let the parietals float back into place and recheck by palpation.

Figure 35: Parietal lift

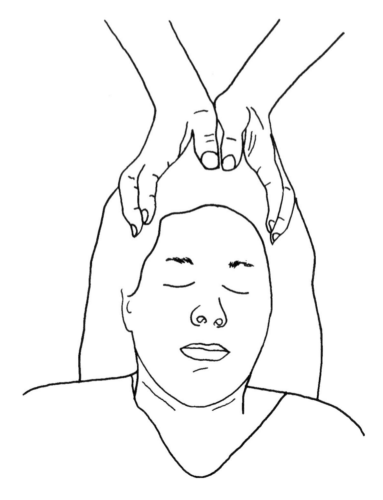

Horizontal Intracranial Membrane Release: Tentorium Cerebelli

Practice: Sphenoid Lift
(Anterior-Posterior Cranial Membrane Traction)

The sphenoid plays a significant role in craniosacral dynamics. It is the keystone of the cranial dynamic system, relates the neurocranium to the face and palate, is integral to vision and smell, and not insignificantly, contains the pituitary, which it rocks within the sella turcica just above the fulcrum of motion. The clinoid processes of the sphenoid are the anterior attachments of the tentorium cerebellum.

The sphenobasilar unit forms much of the cranial base. Cranial base dysfunctions are generally treated via the sphenoid. The sphenobasilar articulation, a synchondrosis, exhibits six ranges of motion and six classic distortion patterns:

1. flexion-extension fixations
2. sidebending fixations
3. torsion fixations
4. vertical strain fixations
5. lateral strain
6. compression

Upledger discusses the cranial base in detail in his first volume.

To adjust the sphenoid, cradle the head in your hands with your fingers relaxed and spread across the base of the occiput. Your thumbs are up. Contact the greater wings beside the orbits and make contact without pressure. It's surprising how little pressure your contact requires to move the sphenoid. It may help to "magnetize" your thumbs.

Begin by compressing your thumbs toward your hands and with them the sphenoid into the occiput. Remember that this junction is anterior to the foramen magnum. Take your time. Drop in and feel the nature of the sphenobasilar compression for a moment, then begin to lift your thumbs straight anterior (toward the ceiling), tractioning the joint and the tentorium cerebellum via the clinoid processes. Feel the occiput as it sinks into your palms, and allow the membranes to shift. Again, use the weight of the head to make the correction. Now test the joint for flexion and extension by passive palpation, and sidebending, torsion, lateral strain, and vertical strain by subtle motion palpation as well. When you push the sphenoid into each range of motion, you are feeling for ease of compliance, elasticity. The joint is not dramatically moveable. Think of it as the meeting of two three-dimensional vectors as you test it.

Figure 36: Sphenoid lift

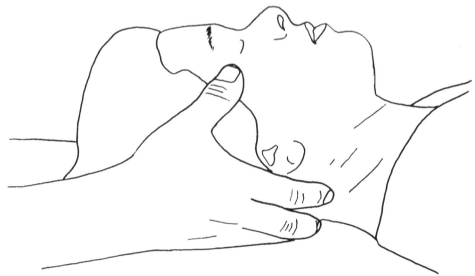

After you have palpated the range of motion (mobility and motility) and distortion patterns of the sphenoid and occiput, drop your attention in to the sphenobasilar joint inside the head and check each range of motion both into and out of distortion to see if there is any inherent motion in there, much as you did at the body diaphragms. If you feel the urge to move, follow it through, becoming immovable in response to any backtracking. When you are satisfied that a shift has occurred, let the joint ease back to normal and recheck by palpation.

Practice: Temporal Ear Pull (Transverse Cranial Membrane Traction)

The temporals contain the auditory and labyrinthine mechanisms and serve as lateral anchors for the transverse tentorium cerebellum, which reaches across the head in tensile harmony with the corpus callosum. The rhythmic influence on the vestibular apparatus is probably significant. Remember that the vestibular system communicates via the endolymphatic sac through a membrane window to the cranial dura.

Place the hands over the parietals and temporals with two fingers on either side of each ear and your fifth fingers pointing down toward the mastoids. Palpate the temporals as they rock forth and back, out and in. The temporals often express compression of the hemispheres, and you can pull them apart using the ears as handles. Grab the lobes lightly with your thumbs and forefingers, diagonally behind and below the auditory meatus. Traction posterior, inferior,

Figure 37: Temporals and labyrinths

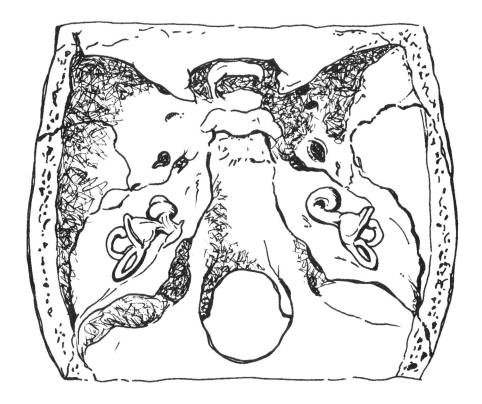

and apart. After you feel the sutures relax, continue your traction down the auditory tube and across the brain. If you feel like allowing some rotation, go ahead. You may feel like torquing the right ear anterior and inferior and pulling straight superior on the left one. Move slowly. Become immovable in response to any backtracking. Allow the membranes to shift. Recheck by palpation.

Figure 38: Temporal ear pull

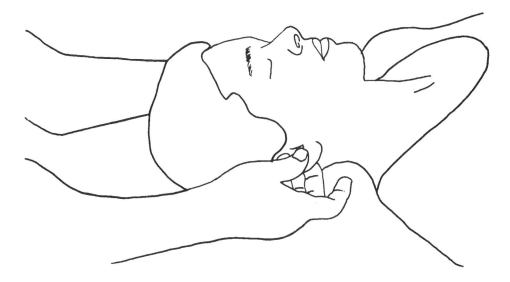

Temporal Rock

"Ride" the rhythm on the temporals for a minute. Is their range the same and are they in sync? Then, at the extreme of either phase of the CRI, hold one side in place and become immovable to it while allowing the other side to move in its natural rhythm. In so splitting the temporal function, you are among other things creating a fulcrum of torsional sagittal motion at the approximate location of the diaphragma sellae, which tents the pituitary. Rock the temporals like this several times. You can hold the extreme ranges for a moment and allow tension to build up a bit before relaxing your hold and torquing the other way. Then again hold one side in one phase and let the other one catch up, returning it to its physiologic motion. Because this adjustment is more interventionist than some of the others, be sure to ride with the normal motion for several cycles, being sure to let the mechanism down lightly so as not to create an iatrogenic fixation in this significant structure.

Finish the adjustment with induction of a still point on the cranium or even at the feet. Recheck by palpation.

Figure 39: Temporal rock

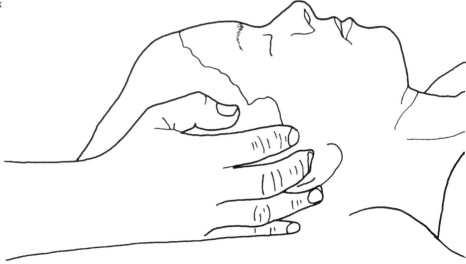

The Ten-Step Protocol

The ten-step protocol was formatted by John Upledger for the purposes of teaching the basics. It covers a lot of territory and is an effective basic treatment procedure as you teach yourself to work with the craniosacral system. As your skills develop, and you naturally abandon the ten-step in favor of a more intuitive, unformatted treatment, the elements of the ten-step will remain ever at your fingertips.

The basis of the ten-step protocol is your palpation. Sit down, place your hands at your station, and listen.

1. Still point induction
2. Transverse diaphragm releases:
    a. Pelvic diaphragm release
    b. Thoracic diaphragm release
    c. Thoracic inlet release
    d. Occipital decompression and dural tube traction
3. Frontal lift
4. Parietal lift
5. Temporal ear pull
6. Temporal rock
7. Sphenoid lift
8. Mandibular decompression
9. Sacral decompression and dural tube traction
10. Still point induction

Chiropractic, Osteopathy, and Medicine

*T*he craniosacral concept is derived directly from osteopathy, which originated in 1874 with Andrew Taylor Still. His contemporary, D.D. Palmer, developed chiropractic beginning in 1895, when a spinal adjustment he delivered to Harvey Lillard instantly restored Lillard's hearing. Still and his school believed that it was the stimulation of spinal vasomotor reflexes, leading to an increase in blood perfusion to the tissues, that was basic to the healing process. Palmer's view was that "nerve energy" itself, raw and pure, provided the impetus for this most valuable transformation. Both men comprehended the spine and both men shared the certainty that healing was inherent and could be encouraged to manifest. Both men resisted the notions of "scientific medicine," and those of each other.

The two schools developed in parallel, both outside of the allopathic medical establishment. In the 1960s they were each approached by the medical hierarchy and offered a chance to "join up," on dictated terms. The osteopaths were offered a better status than the chiropractors and decided by majority to accept membership on these terms. Chiropractors, offered a more limited scope of practice, and one subservient to the abhorrent ideas of pharmacological medicine, denounced the whole business as a blatant attempt to usurp the philosophical momentum that was its birthright. Animosity flared and war was declared. As evidence that the charges of professional sabotage were accurate, osteopathy has evolved into a profession that today remains divided philosophically and politically, and for the most part, scarcely resembles its original form. Because of osteopathy's near-establishment status, the initials D.O. became coveted by those with the ambition to become a medical doctor but lacking the eligibility, for one reason or another, to qualify for medical school.

Today a healthy percentage of the osteopathic profession practices competent family medicine, emergency medicine, and surgery, and for decades a small, proud, and dedicated minority of manipulative osteopaths has more or less quietly suffered the under-the-breath ridicule of their own peers. The cranial concept has been a special target of scorn by whole generations of osteopathic students, and yet the field has continually attracted a core of faithful who have championed and developed the manipulative tradition in osteopathy for a hundred years.

With osteopathy (and naturopathy, another mosquito on the biceps of allopathic medicine) now properly contained, and homeopathy having been vanquished before the time of this story, chiropractic, being more aggressive and defiant than dentists (originally the great nutritionists) and podiatrists, now moved into first place on the enemies list of organized medicine. Such is the way of a civilized and orderly society. Some of allopathic medicine's claims were true, and others were well-intentioned but based in mistrust and misunderstanding, and some were vicious lies. Chiropractors fought back "tooth and nail," and despite all odds have maintained and guarded the niche of the manipulative physician in American society. It is certainly a victory of the common man.

Chiropractic today also remains a profession unified neither philosophically nor politically. The position of chiropractic in the fragile economic ecosystem remains somewhat precarious, but it will certainly survive and continue to prosper. It's likely that the survival of chiropractic owes more to its clinical efficacy than to the articulation of its concepts.

One of the advantages of osteopathy's embracing of allopathic medicine as its overlord has been its privilege in associating, however loosely, with several large universities, therefore keeping the osteopaths in at least potential contact with other disciplines. The university medical school format has led to the natural filtering of osteopathic concepts through unrelated disciplines, like pathology, biochemistry, physics, and engineering. For fifty years, osteopathy has benefitted and continues to benefit from this association. The chiropractic profession, on the other hand, for too long scorned all scientific method, and in return was harassed and discouraged from accredited education. Chiropractic retreated underground, left to communicate amongst itself in the semi-cultlike manner of an isolated caste. It has developed almost entirely in the private sector, isolated from the stimulatory interaction of universities and hospitals, and the opportunities they provide. The more brilliant innovators in chiropractic, inspired with almost evangelical fervor, tended to attract loyal but isolated followings of philosophically eager proponents and were likely to consider any intellectual challenge as a declaration of war.

The battles among the fiefdoms of chiropractic technique have tended to be heated and serious, with the various groups often trying to influence lawmakers into outlawing their internal "enemies." While the controversies in chiropractic have made it a diverse and many-petaled bloom, the discord in chiropractic has had a somewhat less favorable effect. Yet it must be seen as an appanage of the clinical hostility and economic isolation foisted upon it by powerful special interests. That chiropractic has survived and developed in the face of these odds is a testimony to its efficacy and spirit. It has preserved the role of the structural and functional doctor in our society.

As a full-time chiropractor and part-time student of osteopathic concepts, I have been impressed by some of the insights that the many fine minds in the osteopathic profession have revealed about the function of the human organism. Perhaps in the near future we will have the opportunity to contribute some of chiropractic's "great concepts" to that profession, and increasingly to the world at large. The public needs a more unified concept, and a good one. It seems likely that in communicating we will at times be required to rephrase our concepts so that the others can more readily comprehend the essence of our offering. Chiropractic itself can only benefit.

The medical hierarchy seems likely to be headed for a shift, dictated by necessity as health care continues in its present manner. It won't fall but a window will open. Chiropractors, osteopaths, acupuncturists, and even presently unlicensed disciplines will at least have an outside chance to prove ourselves in the mainstream marketplace, barring, perhaps, the socialization of health care. The individual of our society needs a deeper understanding of the mechanisms inherent to his or her functional downfall. It requires from us a faithful adherence to the moral principle typified by the Hippocratic Oath, a primary dedication to service. It also demands that we be the experts in the natural sciences of clinical anatomy and functional (clinical) physiology. This is the niche that by and large remains unfilled in America. Whoever fills it will ultimately succeed because the individual will inherently choose them.

Bibliography

Barr, Murray L., and Kiernan, John A. *The Human Nervous System: An Anatomical Viewpoint.* Philadelphia: Harper & Row, 1983.

Bennett, Terrence J., D.C. *A New Clinical Approach to the Correction of Abnormal Function.* Privately published, 1960.

Berk, *William R. Chinese Healing Arts.* Peace Press, 1979.

Brantingham, James W., D.C. "Dr. Palmer and Dr. Still: The Impact of the First Chiropractor and the First Osteopath." *Chiropractic History,* Volume 6. The Association for the History of Chiropractic, 4920 Frankford Ave. Baltimore, MD: 21206

Breig, Alf. *Adverse Mechanical Tension in the Central Nervous System: An Analysis of Cause and Effect.* New York: John Wiley & Sons,1978.

Carpenter, Malcolm B. Core *Text of Neuroanatomy.* Baltimore: Williams & Wilkins, 1985.

Chusid, Joseph G. *Correlative Neuroanatomy and Functional Neurology.* Los Altos, CA: Lange, 1985.

Cottam, Nephi, D.C., and Calvin, D.C. *Craniopathy For You.* Privately published, 1963.

Cserr, Helen F. *Fluid Environment of the Brain.* New York: Academic Press, 1975.

Davson, Hugh. *Physiology of the Cerebrospinal Fluid.* London: J.A Churchill Ltd., 1967.

DeJarnette, M.B., D.C. *SOT Cranial Manual.* Privately published, 1979.

FitzGerald, M.J.T. *Neuroanatomy Basic & Applied.* London: Bailliere Tindall,1985.

Freud, Sigmund. *The Basic Writings of Sigmund Freud.* Edited by Dr. A.A. Brill. New York: Random House, 1938.

Frymann, Viola M., D.O., F.A.A.O. "Palpation: Its Study In The Workshop." Yearbook reprint. Academy of Applied Osteopathy, 1963.

Gilman and Newman. *Manter & Gatz's Essentials of Clinical Neuroanatomy & Neurophysiology.* Philadelphia: F.A. Davis Co.,1987.

Ganong, W.F. *Review of Medical Physiology,* 9th Edition. Los Altos, CA: Lange Medical Publications, 1979.

Goodheart, George, D.C. *You'll Be Better: The Story of Applied Kinesiology.* Geneva, OH: AK Printing, 1987.

Grossinger, Richard. *Planet Medicine.* Berkeley, CA: North Atlantic Books, 1995.

Guyton, Arthur C. *Textbook of Medical Physiology.* Philadelphia: W.B. Saunders Co., 1976.

Jeannerod, Marc. *The Brain Machine: The Development of Neurophysiological Thought.* Cambridge: Harvard University Press, 1985.

Katzman, Robert, and Pappius, Hanna M. *Brain Electrolytes and Fluid Metabolism.* Baltimore: Williams & Wilkins, 1973.

Keele, Cyril A., and Neil, Eric. *Samson Wright's Applied Physiology.* London: Oxford University Press, 1971.

Keleman, Stanley. *Emotional Anatomy.* Berkeley, CA: Center Press, 1985.

Korr, Irwin M. *The Collected Papers of Irwin M. Korr.* Newark, OH: American Academy of Osteopathy, 1979.

MacDonald, Richard C., D.O., F.A.A.O. Personal communication. 1987.

Magoun, Harold I. *Osteopathy in the Cranial Field.* Kirksville, MO: The Journal Printing Company, 1976.

Milne, Hugh. *The Heart of Listening.* Berkeley, CA: North Atlantic Books, 1995.

Mindell, Arnold. *Dreambody: The Body's Role in Revealing the Self.* New York: Routledge & Kegan Paul, 1984.

Mindell, Arnold. *Working With the Dreaming Body.* New York: Routledge & Kegan Paul, 1985.

Palmer, D.D. *The Chiropractor's Adjuster.* Portland, OR: Portland Printing House Company, 1910.

Pappenheimer, John J. "The Sleep Factor." *Science* (Feb. 1980): vol. 24–30.

Porkert, Manfred. *The Theoretical Foundations of Chinese Medicine.* Cambridge, England: MIT Press, 1974.

Rapoport, Stanley I. *The Blood Brain Barrier in Physiology and Medicine.* New York: Raven Press, 1977.

Editors of Scientific American. *The Physics and Chemistry of Life.* New York: Simon and Schuster, 1955.

Selye, Hans, M.D. *The Stress of Life.* McGraw-Hill, 1978.

Spears, Leo L., D.C. *Spears Painless System.* Denver, CO: Privately published, 1950.

Speransky, A.D. *A Basis For the Theory of Medicine.* New York: International Publishers, 1943.

Still, Andrew T. *Philosophy of Osteopathy.* (1899) Colorado Springs, CO: American Academy of Osteopathy, 1977.

Sutherland, Adah Strand. *With Thinking Fingers*. Kansas City, MO: The Cranial Academy, 1962.

Sutherland, William G. *The Cranial Bowl*. Mankato, MN: Free Press Co., 1948.

Upledger, John E., and Vredevoogd, Jon D. *Craniosacral Therapy*. Chicago: Eastland Press, 1983.

Upledger, John E. *Craniosacral Therapy II: Beyond the Dura*. Seattle: Eastland Press, 1987.

Upledger, John E., *Your Inner Physician and You*. Berkeley, CA: North Atlantic Books, 1993.

Upledger, John E., Personal communication. 1984–1990.

Veith, Ilza. *The Yellow Emperor's Classic of Internal Medicine*. Berkeley: University of California Press, 1949.

Ward, Lowell D.C., PhD, and Koren, Tedd, D.C. "Spinal Column Stressology." *The American Chiropractor* Vol. (July 1987).

Warwick, Roger, and Williams, Peter L. *Gray's Anatomy,* 35th British edition. Philadelphia: W.B. Saunders Co., 1973.

Wilkinson, J.L. *Neuroanatomy For Medical Students*. John Wright & Sons Ltd., 1986.

Wurtman, Richard J. *Nutrition and The Brain*. New York: Raven Press, 1977.

Index